D0966711

The Ethics of
Human Cloning

The Ethics of Human Cloning

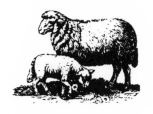

Leon R. Kass
and
James Q. Wilson

The AEI Press
Publisher for the American Enterprise Institute
WASHINGTON, D.C.
1998

Available in the United States from the AEI Press, c/o Publisher
Resources Inc., 1224 Heil Quaker Blvd., P.O. Box 7001, La Vergne,
TN 37086-7001. To order, call toll free: 1-800-269-6267. Distributed
outside the United States by arrangement with Eurospan, 3 Henrietta
Street, London WC2E 8LU, England.

Library of Congress Cataloging-in-Publication Data

Kass, Leon.
    The ethics of human cloning / Leon R. Kass and James Q. Wilson.
        p. cm.
    Includes bibliographical references.
    ISBN 0-8447-4050-0 (alk. paper)
    1. Cloning—Moral and ethical aspects. 2. Human reproductive
technology—Moral and ethical aspects. I. Wilson, James Q.
II. Title.
QH442.2.K37 1998
174 '.25—dc21   98-18223
                                                    CIP

    5 7 9 10 8 6 4

THE AEI PRESS
Publisher for the American Enterprise Institute
1150 17th Street, N.W., Washington, D.C. 20036

Printed in the United States of America

Contents

Introduction

*I*n 1971 James D. Watson, codiscoverer with Francis Crick of the double-helical structure of DNA, predicted that one day human cloning would be possible and urged that "as many people as possible be informed about the new ways for human reproduction and their potential consequences, both good and bad."[1] Watson's prediction seemed far-fetched at the time, and his admonition was ignored. In the subsequent quarter-century, genetics became a booming, rapidly progressing science. Along with prodigious advances in our knowledge of biological nature and many tangible improvements in medical diagnostics and practice, molecular biology generated a series of discrete ethical and policy issues. Does genetic research present public health hazards? Should genetically engineered molecules, tissues, and animals be patentable? Should individuals have a "right to privacy"

---

1. James D. Watson, "Moving toward the Clonal Man," *The Atlantic Monthly,* May 1971, at 50–53.

concerning genetic information (such as predisposition to disease)? Yet the prospect of cloning whole animals, and *Homo sapiens* himself, remained remote, and the ethical implications of such an astounding development went largely unexplored.

That all changed on February 23, 1997, with the news that Dolly the lamb had been cloned from the nonreproductive tissue of one adult female sheep so that she was genetically identical to her sole progenitor.[2] The news was called "extraordinary," "stupendous," "mind-boggling," "frightening," and even "the scientific discovery of the century." Suddenly, Dr. Ian Wilmut, head of the research team at the Roslin Institute in Edinburgh, Scotland, where the cloning took place, went from being an obscure embryologist to the focus of media attention and investor interest. Dolly became a celebrity, the butt of countless jokes, a symbol of modern science, and a source of hype and even hysteria. Most of the commentary, however, was concerned not with Dolly herself or with Dr. Wilmut's scientific discovery, but rather with the specter of human cloning and its implications for human welfare.

---

2. I. Wilmut, A. E. Schnieke, J. McWhir, A. J. Kind, and K. H. S. Campbell, "Viable Offspring Derived from Fetal and Adult Mammalian Cells," 385 *Nature* 810 (February 27, 1997).

In the public debate that followed, two essays stood out for their moral clarity and seriousness regarding "new ways for human reproduction and their potential consequences, both good and bad." James Q. Wilson's "The Paradox of Cloning" (*The Weekly Standard*, May 26, 1997) and Leon Kass's "The Wisdom of Repugnance" (*The New Republic*, June 2, 1997) approached the ethics of human cloning from somewhat different perspectives and came to decidedly different conclusions. Each, however, transcended the initial commentaries on all sides of the issue, and each seems likely to endure as the human cloning debate develops. The American Enterprise Institute reprints the essays here (with a few minor revisions) with the kind permission of their original publishers. Professors Kass and Wilson have both prepared brief additional essays—each commenting on the other's original essay and elaborating his own views—which are published here for the first time. This introduction provides a bit of background about the science of Dolly's cloning and the ensuing debates.

Why Dolly Is Different

Dolly grew from a sheep embryo that had been created not in the usual way—from a female egg joining with a male sperm to produce a genetically mixed offspring—but rather

from an egg that had been implanted with the full comple-
ment of genetic material from a second (female) sheep. Dr.
Wilmut's research group began with a culture of mammary cells drawn from a six-year-old ewe. The cells were
grown in a nutrient-poor culture medium that forced them
into a quiescent state, known as the G0 phase of the cell
cycle (a phase all cells go through in the process of divid-
ing). The researchers then took unfertilized egg cells, called
oocytes, from other ewes and removed each oocyte's
nucleus, leaving the cell wall intact. They then fused the
mammary cells with the enucleated oocytes by bringing
them together and subjecting them to a pulsed electric current—a procedure that stimulated the genetic material from
the mammary cells to act as if it were inside a normal embryo. Of 277 fused cells produced in that manner, 29 sur-
vived longer than a few days and were implanted in the
wombs of thirteen sheep. Only one was carried to term
and born as a live lamb.

The genetic manipulation that produced Dolly is collo-
quially called "cloning." Cloning, however, is a general
term, describing any procedure that produces a precise genetic replica of a biological object, including a DNA se-
quence, a cell, or an organism. Scientists have been cloning
elementary substances such as genes and cells for years; today, much routine biological research and many important

pharmaceutical applications depend on that sort of cloning, which involves few of the ethical dilemmas presented by the cloning of human beings and higher animals.

The procedure that produced Dolly is more precisely termed "somatic cell nuclear transfer" because it involves the transfer of the nucleus of a somatic cell (any cell other than eggs or sperm, which are called germ cells) into an unfertilized egg cell that has had its own nucleus removed. Before Dolly, biologists believed that once somatic cells have become differentiated—that is, have developed from embryonic cells into specialized cells such as those in the muscle or skin—the process of differentiation cannot be reversed. But Dr. Wilmut's research team appears to have demonstrated that this central assumption is incorrect: they "reprogrammed" a fully differentiated (mammary) cell, causing it to behave like an undifferentiated cell and restarting the process of differentiation and growth (a process analogous to rebooting a computer when it is running a specialized application program).[3]

---

3. The report of the National Bioethics Advisory Commission, *Cloning Human Beings* (June 1997), mentioned later in this introduction, contains an excellent account of the science of cloning and somatic cell nuclear transfer, along with extended discussion of religious, ethical, and policy issues presented by human cloning.

That differentiated cells may be returned to their undifferentiated state is what makes it possible to envision cloning fully grown, higher species as well as individual cells and other elementary organisms—thereby giving rise to the ethical issues presented by human cloning. It is important to recognize, however, that Dr. Wilmut's discovery, in addition to being tentative (as are all new and unconfirmed discoveries) may be limited in ways that eliminate or ameliorate the ethical dilemmas. One of the keys to his success, for example, appears to have been arresting the mammary cells in the G0 phase of the cell cycle. If that proves to be the key, cloning will be possible only in those organisms whose cells can be arrested in the G0 phase. Previous attempts to clone mice failed when arresting murine cells in the G0 stage proved all but impossible.

Another factor that may prove critical to the success of cloning sheep is the biochemical environment inside ovine cells. Scientists postulate that this environment gives genetic material from the adult cell at least two rounds of cell division during which it can reprogram itself. But the cells of different organisms have different chemical environments and develop differently at the molecular level; we know that organisms other than sheep do not have such a long grace period in which their genetic material can undifferentiate. Success in cloning a sheep does not guarantee success in cloning other organisms.

Ian Wilmut himself has been careful to point out how little we know about the scientific implications of somatic cell nuclear transfer. He has doubted whether all types of adult cells could be undifferentiated. "Brain and muscle cells are probably so [specialized] that you can't reset their clocks," he has said. He has also noted that species differ in the mechanisms that regulate early development and that those influence the response to nuclear transfer. Pig embryos are different from sheep and cow embryos in that respect, so their response to attempts to clone them may be different.

Another question yet to be answered is whether cells from a very old donor would work. The random genetic mutations that occur over time in living cells—the vast majority of them deleterious—may well prove impossible for an egg to reverse. It remains to be seen whether Dolly will live as long as a normal sheep. Having been produced from a six-year-old cell, she may exhibit signs of aging prematurely. Since techniques of manipulating DNA, such as cloning, sometimes damage DNA (witness Wilmut's 276 failures), Dolly could develop any number of genetically based diseases that could shorten her life.

Genetic variation can start to occur the minute a cell

undergoes cell division. Until recently, scientists believed that when a cell divided to become two cells, the two cells were identical, or clones of each other. We now know that cell replication does not always produce identical copies of the cell. So although much has been made of Dolly's being genetically identical to her progenitor, uncertainty enters the biological equation. Organisms that start life as genetically identical can exhibit very different patterns of protein production, for example.

We also know that even a cloned organism such as Dolly does not inherit *all* its DNA from its progenitor; a small amount of mitochondrial DNA is bequeathed to it by the enucleated oocyte (that is, by the contributor of the egg). Mitochondrial DNA is not located in the nucleus, but in the cytoplasm of a cell. It codes for a number of metabolic proteins and is passed down exclusively through the female of a species. When we talk about cloning an organism of either sex, we must remember that the cloned organism will not inherit its mitochondrial DNA from its progenitor unless its progenitor also donates the oocyte. That means that males cannot be perfectly cloned, and females can be perfectly cloned only if the somatic cell and oocyte come from the same individual—that is, the individual being cloned also provides the egg. We have yet to learn what effect the presence of noncloned mitochondrial DNA has on a cloned organism's development.

Perhaps the biggest factor of uncertainty is the effect that environment has on the development of an organism. We have noted that mitochondrial DNA and variations in the intrauterine environment would produce a cloned offspring somewhat different from its progenitor. But other opportunities for variation, many of them poorly understood, exist. As a complex multicellular organism such as a mammal develops, prenatal and early natal environmental conditions will influence its maturation and can have a significant impact on its development.

Social and Political Responses to Dolly

The first effect of the Dolly announcement was to fire the public imagination. Commentators were quick to speculate about the possibility of cloning a human. The *Los Angeles Times* opined that such a discovery "opens the door to a 'Blade Runner' world of human replicants." No less sober a publication than the *Wall Street Journal* asked business leaders and newsmakers whether they would like to have themselves cloned. Feminists observed that the technique finally made men superfluous. Tabloid newspapers warned of "master races" and promised production lines of movie and sports stars.

Government reaction to the news was swift. President Clinton ordered that no federal funds be spent on human cloning (as far as anyone knows, none had been) and directed the National Bioethics Advisory Commission (NBAC) to "conduct a thorough review of the legal and the ethical issues raised" by human cloning.

The NBAC issued its report, *Cloning Human Beings*, on June 9, 1997. The commission's main conclusion was unequivocal: "At this time it is morally unacceptable for anyone in the public or private sector, whether in a research or clinical setting, to attempt to create a child using somatic cell nuclear transfer cloning."[4] The commission's consensus on that point was based on safety—that is, that using somatic cell nuclear transfer for the purpose of creating a child entailed significant uncertainties and "unacceptable risks to the fetus and/or potential child"—but it also emphasized that "many other serious ethical concerns have been identified, which require much more widespread and careful public deliberation before this technology may be

---

4. *Id*. at iii.

used." At the same time, the commission recognized that somatic cell nuclear transfer technology may have many beneficial applications for biotechnology, livestock production, and new medical applications, including the production of pharmaceutical proteins and prospects for regeneration and repair of human tissues, and it noted that it is "notoriously difficult to draft legislation at any particular moment that can serve to both exploit and govern the rapid and unpredictable advances of science."

The NBAC made the following five recommendations. First, the president's moratorium on the use of federal funds to support any attempt to create a child by somatic cell nuclear transfer should be continued, and all firms, clinicians, investigators, and professional societies should be requested to comply voluntarily with the intent of the federal moratorium. Second, federal legislation should be enacted to prohibit anyone from attempting, whether in a research or clinical setting, to create a child through somatic cell nuclear transfer. Third, the United States should cooperate with other countries to enforce mutually supported restrictions on human cloning. Fourth, any regulatory or legislative actions undertaken to effect a prohibition on human cloning should be carefully written so as not to interfere with other important areas of research, such as the cloning of human DNA sequences and cells. Finally, cloning animals by somatic cell nuclear transfer should be subject only to existing regulations regarding the humane use of animals, since the technique does not raise the same issues implicated in attempting to use it to create a child.

Following release of the NBAC report, President Clinton endorsed legislation to prohibit for five years the use of somatic cell nuclear transfer cloning to create a human being and to continue the ban on the use of federal funds for research leading to human cloning. In 1997 and 1998 numerous bills to ban human cloning were introduced in the U.S. Congress. Most were similar to the version endorsed by the president—banning (temporarily or indefinitely) any effort to use somatic cell nuclear transfer to clone a human being, protecting other forms of genetic research (including the cloning of nonhuman animals), and calling for further study and reports by the NBAC and other bodies.

The scientists, ethicists, religious leaders, and business executives testifying before Congress in hearings on those bills were in general agreement about human cloning. In his testimony before the Senate, Dr. Wilmut said that human cloning would be "unethical" and "quite inhumane." James Geraghty, president of Genzyme Transgenics Corporation, testified that the biotechnology industry overwhelmingly agreed that there is no legitimate reason in our society to clone human beings and stated that biotechnology firms are well aware of the need to operate within socially accepted norms of behavior. Scientists and biotechnology executives were equally insistent, however, that any legal restriction on human cloning avoid interfering with beneficial applications of cloning technologies, such as to produce genetically identical research animals for improving the speed and accuracy of pharmaceutical research. And many witnesses emphasized the numerous uncertainties concerning somatic cell nuclear transfer and the distant prospects of human cloning. Thomas H. Murray of the Center for Biomedical Ethics, for example, emphasized in his testimony before the House of Representatives that "good ethics begins with good facts" and proceeded to describe many of the biological conundrums mentioned earlier in this introduction.

As this book goes to press in the spring of 1998, no national legislation concerning human cloning has been enacted in the United States. (Some restrictions have been enacted in the state of California and in Europe.) But no one doubts that the political debate will continue and intensify—perhaps prompted by further, currently unanticipated scientific developments—and that the likelihood of some form of legislative response is strong.

The issues of scientific uncertainty and legal interference with uncontroversial (or less controversial) forms of genetic research, which have dominated legislative deliberations up to the present, are certainly important aspects of any serious consideration of the ethics of human cloning. The essays presented in this volume, however, proceed directly to the larger question: If human cloning does become a practical reality, is it a reality we humans should countenance? Leon R. Kass and James Q. Wilson share a fundamental aversion to the notion of human cloning, but their reticence derives from different views of the importance of sexual reproduction, the role of the family, and the likely social consequences of human cloning. Professor Kass argues that in vitro fertilization and other assisted reproductive technologies that place "the origin of human life literally in human hands" have led "to the continuing erosion of respect for the mystery of sexuality and human renewal." In his view, permitting human cloning would be a drastic further step in the weakening of human respect for the profundity of sexual union and would lead to the replacement of procreation by manufacturing. Professor Wilson, in contrast, argues that the biology of conception is largely incidental: "cloning presents no special ethical risks if society does all in its power to establish that the child is born to a married woman and is the joint responsibility of the married couple." In his view, with proper social (including legal) protections and support for the institution of marriage, cloning could be, like in vitro fertilization and surrogate motherhood, a limited, beneficial, and ethically untroubling practice for infertile married couples.

Both authors understand that the issue of human cloning is important not only in its own right but as an extension and dramatization of many other, exigent social questions. We hope that their essays will stimulate and deepen the public discussion of the ethics of human cloning and of broader contemporary issues concerning marriage, family, and sexuality as well.

Clarisa Long
Abramson Fellow

Christopher DeMuth
President

American Enterprise Institute
for Public Policy Research

The Ethics of
Human Cloning

Part One

The Wisdom of Repugnance

Leon R. Kass

Our habit of delighting in news of scientific and technological breakthroughs has been sorely challenged by the birth announcement of a sheep named Dolly. Though Dolly shares with previous sheep the "softest clothing, woolly, bright," William Blake's question, "Little Lamb, who made thee?" has for her a radically different answer: Dolly was, quite literally, made. She is the work not of nature or nature's God but of man, an Englishman, Ian Wilmut, and his fellow scientists. What is more, Dolly came into being not only asexually—ironically, just like "He [who] calls Himself a Lamb"—but also as the genetically identical copy (and the perfect incarnation of the form or blueprint) of a mature ewe, of whom she is a clone. This long-awaited yet not quite expected success in cloning a mammal raised immediately the prospect—and the specter—of cloning human beings: "I a child and Thou a lamb," despite our differences, have always been equal candidates for creative making, only now, by means of cloning, we may both spring from the hand of man playing at being God.

After an initial flurry of expert comment and public consternation, with opinion polls showing overwhelming opposition to cloning human beings, President Clinton ordered a ban on all federal support for human cloning research (even though none was being supported) and charged the National Bioethics Advisory Commission to report in ninety days on the ethics of human cloning research. The commission (an eighteen-member panel, evenly balanced between scientists and nonscientists, appointed by the president and reporting to the National Science and Technology Council) invited testimony from scientists, religious thinkers, and bioethicists, as well as from the general public. In its report, issued in June 1997, the commission concluded that attempting to clone a human being was "at this time . . . morally unacceptable," recommended continuing the president's moratorium on the use of federal funds to support cloning of humans, and called for federal legislation to prohibit anyone from attempting (during the next three to five years) to create a child through cloning.

Even before the commission reported, Congress was poised to act. Bills to prohibit the use of federal funds for human cloning research have been introduced in the House of Representatives and the Senate; and another bill, in the House, would make it illegal "for any person to use a human somatic cell for the process of producing a human clone." A fateful decision is at hand. To clone or not to clone a human being is no longer an academic question.

Taking Cloning Seriously, Then and Now

Cloning first came to public attention roughly thirty years ago, following the successful asexual production, in England, of a clutch of tadpole clones by the technique of nuclear transplantation. The individual largely responsible for bringing the prospect and promise of human cloning to public notice was Joshua Lederberg, a Nobel laureate geneticist and a man of large vision. In 1966 Lederberg wrote a remarkable article in the *American Naturalist* detailing the eugenic advantages of human cloning and other forms of genetic engineering, and the following year he devoted a column in the *Washington Post*, where he wrote regularly on science and society, to the prospect of human cloning. He suggested that cloning could help us overcome the unpredictable variety that still rules human reproduction and would allow us to benefit from perpetuating superior genetic endowments. Those writings sparked a small public debate in which I became a participant. At the time a young researcher in molecular biology at the National Institutes of Health, I wrote a reply to the *Post,* arguing against Lederberg's amoral treatment of that morally weighty subject and insisting on the urgency of confronting a series of questions and objections, culminating in the suggestion that "the programmed reproduction of man will, in fact, dehumanize him."

Much has happened in the intervening years. It has become harder, not easier, to discern the true meaning of human cloning. We have in some sense been softened up to the idea—through movies, cartoons, jokes, and intermittent commentary in the mass media, some serious, most lighthearted. We have become accustomed to new practices in human reproduction: not just in vitro fertilization, but also embryo manipulation, embryo donation, and surrogate pregnancy. Animal biotechnology has yielded transgenic animals and a burgeoning science of genetic engineering, easily and soon to be transferable to humans.

Even more important, changes in the broader culture make it now vastly more difficult to express a common and respectful understanding of sexuality, procreation, nascent life, family, and the meaning of motherhood, fatherhood, and the links between the generations. Twenty-five years ago, abortion was still largely illegal and thought to be immoral, the sexual revolution (made possible by the extramarital use of the pill) was still in its infancy, and few had yet heard about the reproductive rights of single women, homosexual men, and lesbians. (Never mind shameless memoirs about one's own incest!) Then one could argue, without embarrassment, that the new technologies of human reproduction—babies without sex—and their confounding of normal kin relations—who is the mother: the egg donor, the surrogate who carries and delivers, or the one who rears?—would "undermine the justification and support that biological parenthood gives to the monogamous marriage." Today, defenders of stable, monogamous marriage risk charges of giving offense to those adults who are living in "new family forms" or to those children who, even without the benefit of assisted reproduction, have acquired either three or four parents or one or none at all. Today, one must even apologize for voicing opinions that twenty-five years ago were nearly universally regarded as the core of our culture's wisdom on those matters. In a world whose once-given natural boundaries are blurred by technological change and whose moral boundaries are seemingly up for grabs, it is much more difficult to make persuasive the still compelling case against cloning human beings. As Raskolnikov put it, "Man gets used to everything —the beast!"

Indeed, perhaps the most depressing feature of the discussions that immediately followed the news about Dolly was their ironical tone, their genial cynicism, their moral fatigue: "An Udder Way of Making Lambs" (*Nature*), "Who Will Cash in on Breakthrough in Cloning?" (*Wall Street Journal*), "Is Cloning Baaaaaaaad?" (*Chicago Tribune*). Gone from the scene are the wise and courageous voices of Theodosius Dobzhansky (genetics), Hans Jonas (philosophy), and Paul Ramsey (theology), who, only twenty-five years ago, all made powerful moral arguments against ever cloning a human being. We are now too sophisticated for such argumentation; we would not be caught in public with a strong moral stance, never mind an absolutist one. We are all, or almost all, postmodernists now.

Cloning turns out to be the perfect embodiment of the ruling opinions of our new age. Thanks to the sexual revolution, we are able to deny in practice, and increasingly in thought, the inherent procreative teleology of sexuality itself. But, if sex has no intrinsic connection to generating babies, babies need have no necessary connection to sex. Thanks to feminism and the gay rights movement, we are increasingly encouraged to treat the natural heterosexual difference and its preeminence as a matter of "cultural construction." But if male and female are not normatively complementary and generatively significant, babies need not come from male and female complementarity. Thanks to the prominence and the acceptability of divorce and out-of-wedlock births, stable, monogamous marriage as the ideal home for procreation is no longer the agreed-upon cultural norm. For that new dispensation, the clone is the ideal emblem: the ultimate "single-parent child."

Thanks to our belief that all children should be *wanted* children (the more high-minded principle we use to justify contraception and abortion), sooner or later only those children who fulfill our wants will be fully acceptable. Through cloning, we can work our wants and wills on the very identity of our children, exercising control as never before. Thanks to modern notions of individualism and the rate of cultural change, we see ourselves not as linked to ancestors and defined by traditions, but as projects for our own self-creation, not only as self-made men but also man-made selves; and self-cloning is simply an extension of such rootless and narcissistic self–re-creation.

Unwilling to acknowledge our debt to the past and un-willing to embrace the uncertainties and the limitations of the future, we have a false relation to both: cloning per-sonifies our desire fully to control the future, while being subject to no controls ourselves. Enchanted and enslaved by the glamour of technology, we have lost our awe and wonder before the deep mysteries of nature and of life. We cheerfully take our own beginnings in our hands and, like the last man, we blink.

Part of the blame for our complacency lies, sadly, with the field of bioethics itself, and its claim to expertise in these moral matters. Bioethics was founded by people who understood that the new biology touched and threatened the deepest matters of our humanity: bodily integrity, iden-tity and individuality, lineage and kinship, freedom and self-command, eros and aspiration, and the relations and striv-ings of body and soul. With its capture by analytic philosophy, however, and its inevitable routinization and professionalization, the field has by and large come to con-tent itself with analyzing moral arguments, reacting to new technological developments, and taking on emerging is-sues of public policy, all performed with a naïve faith that the evils we fear can all be avoided by compassion, regulation, and a respect for autonomy. Bioethics has made some major contributions in the protection of human subjects and in other areas where personal freedom is threatened; but its practitioners, with few exceptions, have turned the big human questions into pretty thin gruel.

One reason for that is that the piecemeal formation of public policy tends to grind down large questions of morals into small questions of procedure. Many of the country's leading bioethicists have served on national commissions or state task forces and advisory boards, where, understandably, they have found utilitarianism to be the only ethical vocabulary acceptable to all participants in discussing issues of law, regulation, and public policy. As many of those commissions have been either officially under the aegis of the National Institutes of Health or the Health and Human Services Department, or otherwise dominated by powerful voices for scientific progress, the ethicists have for the most part been content, after some "values clarification" and wringing of hands, to pronounce their blessings upon the inevitable. Indeed, it is the bioethicists, not the scientists, who are now the most articulate defenders of human cloning: the two witnesses testifying before the National Bioethics Advisory Commission in favor of cloning human beings were bioethicists, eager to rebut what they regard as the irrational concerns of those of us in opposition. We have come to expect from the "experts" an accommodationist ethic that will rubber-stamp all biomedical innovation, in the mistaken belief that all other goods must bow down to the gods of better health and scientific advance. Regrettably, as we shall see near the end of this essay, the report of the present commission, though better than its predecessors, is finally not an exception.

If we are to correct our moral myopia, we must first of all persuade ourselves not to be complacent about what is at issue here. Human cloning, though it is in some respects continuous with previous reproductive technologies, also represents something radically new, in itself and in its easily foreseeable consequences. The stakes are very high indeed. I exaggerate, but in the direction of the truth, when I insist that we are faced with having to decide nothing less than whether human procreation is going to remain human, whether children are going to be made rather than begotten, whether it is a good thing, humanly speaking, to say yes in principle to the road that leads (at best) to the dehumanized rationality of *Brave New World*. This is not business as usual, to be fretted about for a while but finally to be given our seal of approval. We must rise to the occasion and make our judgments as if the future of our humanity hangs in the balance. For so it does.

The State of the Art

If we should not underestimate the significance of human cloning, neither should we exaggerate its imminence or misunderstand just what is involved. The procedure is conceptually simple. The nucleus of a mature but unfertilized egg is removed and replaced with a nucleus obtained from a specialized cell of an adult (or fetal) organism (in Dolly's case, the donor nucleus came from mammary gland epithelium). Since almost all the hereditary material of a cell is contained within its nucleus, the renucleated egg and the individual into which that egg develops are genetically identical to the organism that was the source of the transferred nucleus. An unlimited number of genetically identical individuals—clones—could be produced by nuclear transfer. In principle, any person, male or female, newborn or adult, could be cloned, and in any quantity. With laboratory cultivation and storage of tissues, cells outliving their sources make it possible even to clone the dead.

The technical stumbling block, overcome by Wilmut

and his colleagues, was to find a means of reprogramming the state of the DNA in the donor cells, reversing its differentiated expression and restoring its full totipotency, so that it could again direct the entire process of producing a mature organism. Now that the problem has been solved, we should expect a rush to develop cloning for other animals, especially livestock, to propagate in perpetuity the champion meat or milk producers. Though exactly how soon someone will succeed in cloning a human being is anybody's guess, Wilmut's technique, almost certainly applicable to humans, makes *attempting* the feat an imminent possibility.

Yet some cautions are in order and some possible misconceptions need correcting. For a start, cloning is not Xeroxing. As has been reassuringly reiterated, the clone of Mel Gibson, though his genetic double, would enter the world hairless, toothless, and peeing in his diapers, just like any other human infant. Moreover, the success rate, at least at first, will probably not be very high: the British transferred 277 adult nuclei into enucleated sheep eggs and implanted twenty-nine clonal embryos, but they achieved the birth of only one live lamb clone. For that reason, among others, it is unlikely that, at least for now, the practice would be very popular, and there is no immediate worry of mass-scale production of multicopies. The need of repeated surgery to obtain eggs and, more crucially, of numerous borrowed wombs for implantation will surely limit use, as will the expense; besides, almost everyone who is able will doubtless prefer nature's sexier way of conceiving.

Still, for the tens of thousands of people already sustaining over 200 assisted-reproduction clinics in the United States and already availing themselves of in vitro fertilization, intracytoplasmic sperm injection, and other techniques of assisted reproduction, cloning would be an option with virtually no added fuss (especially when the success rate improves). Should commercial interests develop in "nucleus-banking," as they have in sperm-banking; should famous athletes or other celebrities decide to market their DNA the way they now market their autographs and just about everything else; should techniques of embryo and germline genetic testing and manipulation arrive as anticipated, increasing the use of laboratory assistance to obtain "better" babies—should all this come to pass, then cloning, if it is permitted, could become more than a marginal practice simply on the basis of free reproductive choice, even without any social encouragement to upgrade the gene pool or to replicate superior types. Moreover, if laboratory research on human cloning proceeds, even without any intention to produce cloned humans, the existence of cloned human embryos in the laboratory, created to begin with only for research purposes, would surely pave the way for later baby-making implantations.

In anticipation of human cloning, apologists and proponents have already made clear possible uses of the perfected technology, ranging from the sentimental and compassionate to the grandiose. They include: providing a child for an infertile couple; "replacing" a beloved spouse or child who is dying or has died; avoiding the risk of genetic disease; permitting reproduction for homosexual men and lesbians who want nothing sexual to do with the opposite sex; securing a genetically identical source of organs or tissues perfectly suitable for transplantation; getting a child with a genotype of one's own choosing, not excluding oneself; replicating individuals of great genius, talent, or beauty—having a child who really could "be like Mike"; and creating large sets of genetically identical humans suitable for research on, for instance, the question of nature versus nurture, or for special missions in peace and war (not excluding espionage), in which using identical humans would be an advantage. Most people who envision the cloning of human beings, of course, want none of those scenarios. That they cannot say why is not surprising. What is surprising, and welcome, is that, in our cynical age, they are saying anything at all.

The Wisdom of Repugnance

Offensive, grotesque, revolting, repugnant, and *repulsive*—those are the words most commonly heard regarding the prospect of human cloning. Such reactions come both from the man or woman in the street and from the intellectuals, from believers and atheists, from humanists and scientists. Even Dolly's creator has said he "would find it offensive" to clone a human being.

People are repelled by many aspects of human cloning. They recoil from the prospect of mass production of human beings, with large clones of look-alikes, compromised in their individuality; the idea of father-son or mother-daughter twins; the bizarre prospects of a woman's giving birth to and rearing a genetic copy of herself, her spouse, or even her deceased father or mother; the grotesqueness of conceiving a child as an exact replacement for another who has died; the utilitarian creation of embryonic genetic duplicates of oneself, to be frozen away or created when necessary, in case of need for homologous tissues or organs for transplantation; the narcissism of those who would clone themselves and the arrogance of others who think they know who deserves to be cloned or which genotype any child-to-be should be thrilled to receive; the Frank-ensteinian hubris to create human life and increasingly to control its destiny; man playing God. Almost no one finds any of the suggested reasons for human cloning compelling; almost everyone anticipates its possible misuses and abuses. Moreover, many people feel oppressed by the sense that there is probably nothing we can do to prevent it from happening. That makes the prospect all the more revolting.

Revulsion is not an argument; and some of yesterday's repugnances are today calmly accepted—though, one must add, not always for the better. In crucial cases, however, repugnance is the emotional expression of deep wisdom, beyond reason's power fully to articulate it. Can anyone really give an argument fully adequate to the horror which is father-daughter incest (even with consent), or having sex with animals, or mutilating a corpse, or eating human flesh, or raping or murdering another human being? Would anybody's failure to give full rational justification for his revulsion at those practices make that revulsion ethically suspect? Not at all. On the contrary, we are suspicious of

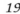

those who think that they can rationalize away our horror, say, by trying to explain the enormity of incest with arguments only about the genetic risks of inbreeding.

The repugnance at human cloning belongs in that category. We are repelled by the prospect of cloning human beings not because of the strangeness or novelty of the undertaking, but because we intuit and feel, immediately and without argument, the violation of things that we rightfully hold dear. Repugnance, here as elsewhere, revolts against the excesses of human willfulness, warning us not to transgress what is unspeakably profound. Indeed, in this age in which everything is held to be permissible so long as it is freely done, in which our given human nature no longer commands respect, in which our bodies are regarded as mere instruments of our autonomous rational wills, repugnance may be the only voice left that speaks up to defend the central core of our humanity. Shallow are the souls that have forgotten how to shudder.

The goods protected by repugnance are generally overlooked by our customary ways of approaching all new biomedical technologies. The way we evaluate cloning ethically will in fact be shaped by how we characterize it descriptively, by the context into which we place it, and by the perspective from which we view it. The first task for ethics is proper description. And here is where our failure begins.

Typically, cloning is discussed in one or more of three familiar contexts, which one might call the technological, the liberal, and the meliorist. Under the first, cloning will be seen as an extension of existing techniques for assisting reproduction and determining the genetic makeup of children. Like them, cloning is to be regarded as a neutral technique, with no inherent meaning or goodness, but subject to multiple uses, some good, some bad. The morality of cloning thus depends absolutely on the goodness or badness of the motives and intentions of the cloners. As one bioethicist defender of cloning puts it, "The ethics must be judged [only] by the way the parents nurture and rear their resulting child and whether they bestow the same love and affection on a child brought into existence by a technique of assisted reproduction as they would on a child born in the usual way."

The liberal (or libertarian or liberationist) perspective sets cloning in the context of rights, freedoms, and personal empowerment. Cloning is just a new option for exercising an individual's right to reproduce or to have the kind of child that he wants. Alternatively, cloning enhances our liberation (especially women's liberation) from the confines of nature, the vagaries of chance, or the necessity for sexual mating. Indeed, it liberates women from the need for men altogether, for the process requires only eggs, nuclei, and (for the time being) uteri—plus, of course, a healthy dose of our (allegedly "masculine") manipulative science that likes to do all those things to mother nature and nature's mothers. For those who hold this outlook, the only moral restraints on cloning are adequately informed consent and the avoidance of bodily harm. If no one is cloned without her consent, and if the clonant is not physically damaged, then the liberal conditions for licit, hence moral, conduct are met. Worries that go beyond violating the will or maiming the body are dismissed as "symbolic"—which is to say, unreal.

The meliorist perspective embraces valetudinarians and also eugenicists. The latter were formerly more vocal in those discussions, but they are now generally happy to see their goals advanced under the less threatening banners of freedom and technological growth. These people see in cloning a new prospect for improving human beings—minimally, by ensuring the perpetuation of healthy individuals by avoiding the risks of genetic disease inherent in the lottery of sex, and maximally, by producing "optimum babies," preserving outstanding genetic material, and (with the help of soon-to-come techniques for precise genetic engineering) enhancing inborn human capacities on many fronts. Here the morality of cloning as a means is justified solely by the excellence of the end, that is, by the outstanding traits of individuals cloned—beauty, or brawn, or brains.

These three approaches, all quintessentially American and all perfectly fine in their places, are sorely wanting as approaches to human procreation. It is, to say the least, grossly distorting to view the wondrous mysteries of birth, renewal, and individuality, and the deep meaning of parent–child relations, largely through the lens of our reductive science and its potent technologies. Similarly, considering reproduction (and the intimate relations of family life!) primarily under the political-legal, adversarial, and individualistic notion of rights can only undermine the private yet fundamentally social, cooperative, and duty-laden character of child-bearing, child-rearing, and their bond to the covenant of marriage. Seeking to escape entirely from nature (to satisfy a natural desire or a natural right to reproduce!) is self-contradictory in theory and self-alienating in practice. For we are erotic beings only because we are embodied beings and not merely intellects and wills unfortunately imprisoned in our bodies. And, though health and fitness are clearly great goods, there is something deeply disquieting in looking on our prospective children as artful products perfectible by genetic engineering, increasingly held to our willfully imposed designs, specifications, and margins of tolerable error.

The technical, liberal, and meliorist approaches all ignore the deeper anthropological, social, and, indeed, ontological meanings of bringing forth a new life. To this more fitting and profound point of view cloning shows itself to be a major violation of our given nature as embodied, gendered, and engendering beings—and of the social relations built on this natural ground. Once this perspective is recognized, the ethical judgment on cloning can no longer be reduced to a matter of motives and intentions, rights and freedoms, benefits and harms, or even means and ends. It must be regarded primarily as a matter of meaning: Is cloning a fulfillment of human begetting and belonging? Or is cloning rather, as I contend, their pollution and perversion? To pollution and perversion the fitting response can only be horror and revulsion; and conversely, generalized horror and revulsion are prima facie evidence of foulness and violation. The burden of moral argument must fall entirely on those who want to declare the widespread repugnances of humankind to be mere timidity or superstition.

Yet repugnance need not stand naked before the bar of reason. The wisdom of our horror at human cloning can be partially articulated, even if this is finally one of those instances about which the heart has its reasons that reason cannot entirely know.

The Profundity of Sex

To see cloning in its proper context, we must begin not, as I did before, with laboratory technique, but with the anthropology—natural and social—of sexual reproduction.

Sexual reproduction—by which I mean the generation of new life from (exactly) two complementary elements, one female, one male, (usually) through coitus—is established (if that is the right term) not by human decision, culture, or tradition, but by nature; it is the natural way of all mammalian reproduction. By nature, each child has two complementary biological progenitors. Each child thus stems from and unites exactly two lineages. In natural generation, moreover, the precise genetic constitution of the resulting offspring is determined by a combination of nature and chance, not by human design: each human child shares the common natural human species genotype, each child is genetically (equally) kin to each (both) parent(s), yet each child is also genetically unique.

Those biological truths about our origins foretell deep truths about our identity and about our human condition altogether. Every one of us is at once equally human, equally enmeshed in a particular familial nexus of origin, and equally individuated in our trajectory from birth to death—and, if all goes well, equally capable (despite our mortality) of participating, with a complementary other, in the very same renewal of such human possibility through procreation. Though less momentous than our common humanity, our genetic individuality is not humanly trivial. It shows itself forth in our distinctive appearance through which we are everywhere recognized; it is revealed in our "signature" marks of fingerprints and our self-recognizing immune system; it symbolizes and foreshadows exactly the unique, never-to-be-repeated character of each human life.

Human societies virtually everywhere have structured child-rearing responsibilities and systems of identity and relationship on the bases of those deep natural facts of begetting. The mysterious yet ubiquitous "love of one's own" is everywhere culturally exploited, to make sure that children are not just produced but well cared for and to create for everyone clear ties of meaning, belonging, and obligation. But it is wrong to treat such naturally rooted social practices as mere cultural constructs (like left- or right-driving, or like burying or cremating the dead) that we can alter with little human cost. What would kinship be without its clear natural grounding? And what would identity be without kinship? We must resist those who have begun to refer to sexual reproduction as the "traditional method of reproduction," who would have us regard as merely traditional, and by implication arbitrary, what is in truth not only natural but most certainly profound.

Asexual reproduction, which produces "single-parent" offspring, is a radical departure from the natural human way, confounding all normal understandings of father, mother, sibling, and grandparent and all moral relations tied thereto. It becomes even more of a radical departure when the resulting offspring is a clone derived not from an embryo, but from a mature adult to whom the clone would be an identical twin; and when the process occurs not by natural accident (as in natural twinning), but by deliberate human design and manipulation; and when the child's (or children's) genetic constitution is preselected by the parent(s) (or scientists). Accordingly, as we shall see, cloning is vulnerable to three kinds of concerns and objections, related to these three points: cloning threatens confusion of identity and individuality, even in small-scale cloning; cloning represents a giant step (though not the first one) toward transforming procreation into manufacture, that is, toward the increasing depersonalization of the process of generation and, increasingly, toward the "production" of human children as artifacts, products of human will and design (what others have called the problem of "commodification" of new life); and cloning—like other forms of eugenic engineering of the next generation—represents a form of despotism of the cloners over the cloned, and thus (even in benevolent cases) represents a blatant violation of the inner meaning of parent-child relations, of what it means to have a child, of what it means to say yes to our own demise and "replacement."

Before turning to those specific ethical objections, let me test my claim of the profundity of the natural way by taking up a challenge recently posed by a friend. What if the given natural human way of reproduction were asexual, and we now had to deal with a new technological innovation—artificially induced sexual dimorphism and the fusing of complementary gametes—whose inventors argued that sexual reproduction promised all sorts of advantages, including hybrid vigor and the creation of greatly increased individuality? Would one then be forced to defend natural asexuality because it was natural? Could one claim that it carried deep human meaning?

The response to that challenge broaches the ontological meaning of sexual reproduction. For it is impossible, I submit, for there to have been human life—or even higher forms of animal life—in the absence of sexuality and sexual reproduction. We find asexual reproduction only in the lowest forms of life: bacteria, algae, fungi, some lower invertebrates. Sexuality brings with it a new and enriched relationship to the world. Only sexual animals can seek and find complementary others with whom to pursue a goal that transcends their own existence. For a sexual being, the world is no longer an indifferent and largely homogeneous *otherness,* in part edible, in part dangerous. It also contains some very special and related and complementary beings, of the same kind but of opposite sex, toward whom one reaches out with special interest and intensity. In higher birds and mammals, the outward gaze keeps a lookout not only for food and predators, but also for prospective mates; the beholding of the many-splendored world is suffused with desire for union—the animal antecedent of human eros and the germ of sociality. Not by accident is the human animal both the sexiest animal—whose females do not go into heat but are receptive throughout the estrous cycle and whose males must therefore have greater sexual appetite and energy to reproduce successfully—and also the most aspiring, the most social, the most open, and the most intelligent animal.

The soul-elevating power of sexuality is, at bottom, rooted in its strange connection to mortality, which it simultaneously accepts and tries to overcome. Asexual reproduction may be seen as a continuation of the activity of self-preservation. When one organism buds or divides to become two, the original being is (doubly) preserved, and nothing dies. Sexuality, by contrast, means perishability and serves replacement; the two that come together to generate one soon will die. Sexual desire, in human beings as in animals, thus serves an end that is partly hidden from, and finally at odds with, the self-serving individual. Whether we know it or not, when we are sexually active we are voting with our genitalia for our own demise. The salmon swimming upstream to spawn and die tell the universal story: sex is bound up with death, to which it holds a partial answer in procreation.

The salmon and the other animals evince that truth blindly. Only the human being can understand what it means. As we learn so powerfully from the story of the Garden of Eden, our humanization is coincident with sexual self-

consciousness, with the recognition of our sexual naked-
ness and all that it implies: shame at our needy incomplete-
ness, unruly self-division, and finitude; awe before the eter-
nal; hope in the self-transcending possibilities of children
and a relationship to the divine. In the sexually self-
conscious animal, sexual desire can become eros, lust can
become love. Sexual desire humanly regarded is thus sub-
limated into erotic longing for wholeness, completion, and
immortality, which drives us knowingly into the embrace
and its generative fruit—as well as into all the higher human possibilities of deed, speech, and song.

Through children, a good common to both husband
and wife, male and female achieve some genuine unifica-
tion (beyond the mere sexual "union," which fails to do
so). The two become one through sharing generous (not
needy) love for that third being as good. Flesh of their flesh,
the child is the parents' own commingled being external-
ized and given a separate and persisting existence. Unifica-
tion is enhanced also by their commingled work of rearing. Providing an opening to the future beyond the grave,
carrying not only our seed but also our names, our ways,
and our hopes that they will surpass us in goodness and
happiness, children are a testament to the possibility of tran-
scendence. Gender duality and sexual desire, which first

draws our love upward and outside of ourselves, finally provide for the partial overcoming of the confinement and limitation of perishable embodiment altogether.

Human procreation, in sum, is not simply an activity of our rational wills. It is a more complete activity precisely because it engages us bodily, erotically, and spiritually as well as rationally. There is wisdom in the mystery of nature that has joined the pleasure of sex, the inarticulate longing for union, the communication of the loving embrace, and the deep-seated and only partly articulate desire for children in the very activity by which we continue the chain of human existence and participate in the renewal of human possibility. Whether or not we know it, the severing of procreation from sex, love, and intimacy is inherently dehumanizing, no matter how good the product.

We are now ready for the more specific objections to cloning.

The Perversities of Cloning

First, an important if formal objection: any attempt to clone a human being would constitute an unethical experiment upon the resulting child-to-be. As the animal experiments (frog and sheep) indicate, there are grave risks of mishaps and deformities. Moreover, because of what cloning means, one cannot presume a future cloned child's consent to be a clone, even a healthy one. Thus, ethically speaking, we cannot even get to know whether or not human cloning is feasible.

I understand, of course, the philosophical difficulty of trying to compare a life with defects against nonexistence. Several bioethicists, proud of their philosophical cleverness, use that conundrum to embarrass claims that one can injure a child in its conception, precisely because it is only thanks to that complained-of conception that the child is alive to complain. But common sense tells us that we have no reason to fear such philosophisms. For we surely know that people can harm and even maim children in the very act of conceiving them, say, by paternal transmission of the AIDS virus, maternal transmission of heroin dependence, or, arguably, even by bringing them into being as bastards or with no capacity or willingness to look after them properly. And we believe that to do that intentionally, or even negligently, is inexcusable and clearly unethical.

The objection about the impossibility of presuming consent may even go beyond the obvious and sufficient point that a clonant, were he subsequently to be asked, could rightly resent having been made a clone. At issue are not just benefits and harms, but doubts about the very independence needed to give proper (even retroactive) consent, that is, not just the capacity to choose but the disposition and ability to choose freely and well. It is not at all clear to what extent a clone will fully be a moral agent. For, as we shall see, in the very fact of cloning, and especially of rearing him *as a clone,* his makers subvert the cloned child's independence, beginning with that aspect that comes from knowing that one was an unbidden surprise, a gift, to the world, rather than the designed result of someone's artful project.

Cloning creates serious issues of identity and individuality. The cloned person may experience concerns about his distinctive identity not only because he will be in genotype and appearance identical to another human being, but, in this case, because he may also be twin to the person who is his "father" or "mother"—if one can still call them that. What would be the psychic burdens of being the "child" or "parent" of your twin? The cloned individual, moreover, will be saddled with a genotype that has already lived. He will not be fully a surprise to the world. People are likely always to compare his performances in life with that of his alter ego. True, his nurture and his circumstance in life will be different; genotype is not exactly destiny. Still, one must also expect parental and other efforts to shape that new life after the original—or at least to view the child with the original version always firmly in mind. Why else did they clone from the star basketball player, mathematician, and beauty queen—or even dear old dad—in the first place?

Since the birth of Dolly, there has been a fair amount of doublespeak on the matter of genetic identity. Experts have rushed in to reassure the public that the clone would in no way be the same person or have any confusions about his identity: as previously noted, they are pleased to point out that the clone of Mel Gibson would not be Mel Gibson. Fair enough. But one is shortchanging the truth by emphasizing the additional importance of the intrauterine environment, rearing, and social setting: genotype obviously matters plenty. That, after all, is the only reason to clone, whether human beings or sheep. The odds that clones of Wilt Chamberlain will play in the NBA are, I submit, infinitely greater than they are for clones of Robert Reich.

Curiously, this conclusion is supported, inadvertently, by the one ethical sticking point insisted on by friends of cloning: no cloning without the donor's consent. Though an orthodox liberal objection, it is in fact quite puzzling when it comes from people (such as Ruth Macklin) who also insist that genotype is not identity or individuality and who deny that a child could reasonably complain about being made a genetic copy. If the clone of Mel Gibson would not be Mel Gibson, why should Mel Gibson have grounds to object that someone had been made his clone? We already allow researchers to use blood and tissue samples for research purposes of no benefit to their sources: my falling hair, my expectorations, my urine, and even my biopsied tissues are "not me" and not mine. Courts have held that the profit gained from uses to which scientists put my discarded tissues do not legally belong to me. Why, then, no cloning without consent—including, I assume, no cloning from the body of someone who just died? What harm is done the donor, if genotype is "not me"? Truth to tell, the only powerful justification for objecting is that genotype really does have something to do with identity, and everybody knows it. If not, on what basis could Michael Jordan object that someone cloned "him," say, from cells taken from a "lost" scraped-off piece of his skin? The insistence on donor consent unwittingly reveals the problem of identity in all cloning.

Genetic distinctiveness not only symbolizes the uniqueness of each human life and the independence of its parents that each human child rightfully attains. It can also be an important support for living a worthy and dignified life.

Such arguments apply with great force to any large-scale replication of human individuals. But they are sufficient, in my view, to rebut even the first attempts to clone a human being. One must never forget that these are human beings upon whom our eugenic or merely playful fantasies are to be enacted.

Troubled psychic identity (distinctiveness), based on all-too-evident genetic identity (sameness), will be made much worse by the utter confusion of social identity and kinship ties. For, as already noted, cloning radically confounds lineage and social relations, for "offspring" as for "parents." As bioethicist James Nelson has pointed out, a female child cloned from her "mother" might develop a desire for a relationship to her "father" and might understandably seek out the father of her "mother," who is after all also her biological twin sister. Would "grandpa," who thought his paternal duties concluded, be pleased to discover that the clonant looked to him for paternal attention and support?

Social identity and social ties of relationship and responsibility are widely connected to, and supported by, biological kinship. Social taboos on incest (and adultery) everywhere serve to keep clear who is related to whom (and especially which child belongs to which parents), as well as to avoid confounding the social identity of parent-and-child (or brother-and-sister) with the social identity of lovers, spouses, and coparents. True, social identity is altered by adoption (but as a matter of the best interest of already living children: we do not deliberately produce children for adoption). True, artificial insemination and in vitro fertilization with donor sperm, or whole embryo donation, are in some way forms of "prenatal adoption"—a not altogether unproblematic practice. Even here, though, there is in each case (as in all sexual reproduction) a known male source of sperm and a known single female source of egg— a genetic father and a genetic mother—should anyone care to know (as adopted children often do) who is genetically related to whom.

In the case of cloning, however, there is but one "parent." The usually sad situation of the "single-parent child" is here deliberately planned, and with a vengeance. In the case of self-cloning, the "offspring" is, in addition, one's twin; and so the dreaded result of incest—to be parent to one's sibling—is here brought about deliberately, albeit without any act of coitus. Moreover, all other relationships will be confounded. What will *father, grandfather, aunt, cousin,* and *sister* mean? Who will bear what ties and what burdens? What sort of social identity will someone have with one whole side—"father's" or "mother's"—necessarily excluded? It is no answer to say that our society, with its high incidence of divorce, remarriage, adoption, extramarital child-bearing, and the rest, already confounds lineage and confuses kinship and responsibility for children (and everyone else), unless one also wants to argue that this is, for children, a preferable state of affairs.

Human cloning would also represent a giant step toward turning begetting into making, procreation into manufacture (literally, something "handmade"), a process already begun with in vitro fertilization and genetic testing of embryos. With cloning, not only is the process in hand, but the total genetic blueprint of the cloned individual is selected and determined by the human artisans. To be sure, subsequent development will take place according to natural processes; and the resulting children will still be recognizably human. But we here would be taking a major step into making man himself simply another one of the man-made things. Human nature becomes merely the last part of nature to succumb to the technological project, which turns all of nature into raw material at human disposal, to be homogenized by our rationalized technique according to the subjective prejudices of the day.

How does begetting differ from making? In natural procreation, human beings come together, complementarily male and female, to give existence to another being who is formed, exactly as we were, *by what we are:* living, hence perishable, hence aspiringly erotic, human beings. In clonal reproduction, by contrast, and in the more advanced forms of manufacture to which it leads, we give existence to a being not by what we are but by what we intend and design. As with any product of our making, no matter how excellent, the artificer stands above it, not as an equal but as a superior, transcending it by his will and creative prowess. Scientists who clone animals make it perfectly clear that they are engaged in instrumental making; the animals are, from the start, designed as means to serve rational human purposes. In human cloning scientists and prospective "parents" would be adopting the same technocratic mentality to human children: human children would be their artifacts.

Such an arrangement is profoundly dehumanizing, no matter how good the product. Mass-scale cloning of the same individual makes the point vividly; but the violation of human equality, freedom, and dignity is present even in a single planned clone. And procreation dehumanized into manufacture is further degraded by commodification, a virtually inescapable result of allowing baby-making to proceed under the banner of commerce. Genetic and reproductive biotechnology companies are already growth industries, but they will go into commercial orbit once the Human Genome Project nears completion. Supply will create enormous demand. Even before the capacity for human cloning arrives, established companies will have invested in the harvesting of eggs from ovaries obtained at autopsy or through ovarian surgery, practiced embryonic genetic alteration, and initiated the stockpiling of prospective donor tissues. Through the rental of surrogate-womb services and through the buying and selling of tissues and embryos, priced according to the merit of the donor, the commodification of nascent human life will be unstoppable.

Finally, and perhaps most important, the practice of human cloning by nuclear transfer—like other anticipated forms of genetic engineering of the next generation—would enshrine and aggravate a profound and mischievous misunderstanding of the meaning of having children and of the parent-child relationship. When a couple now chooses to procreate, the partners are saying yes to the emergence of new life in its novelty, saying yes not only to having a child but also, tacitly, to having whatever child the child turns out to be. In accepting our finitude and opening ourselves to our replacement, we are tacitly confessing the limits of our control. In this ubiquitous way of nature, embracing the future by procreating means precisely that we are relinquishing our grip, in the very activity of taking up our own share in what we hope will be the immortality of human life and the human species. This means that our children are not *our* children: they are not our property, not our possessions. Neither are they supposed to live our lives for us, or anyone else's life but their own. To be sure, we seek to guide them on their way, imparting to them not just life but nurturing, love, and a way of life; to be sure, they bear our hopes that they will live fine and flourishing lives, enabling us in small measure to transcend our own limitations. Still, their genetic distinctiveness and independence are the natural foreshadowing of the deep truth that they have their own and never-before-enacted life to live. They are sprung from a past, but they take an uncharted course into the future.

Much harm is already done by parents who try to live vicariously through their children. Children are sometimes compelled to fulfill the broken dreams of unhappy parents; John Doe, Jr., or John Doe III is under the burden of having to live up to his forebear's name. Still, if most parents have hopes for their children, cloning parents will have expectations. In cloning, such overbearing parents take at the start a decisive step that contradicts the entire meaning of the open and forward-looking nature of parent-child relations. The child is given a genotype that has already lived, with full expectation that the blueprint of a past life ought to be controlling of the life that is to come. Cloning is inherently despotic, for it seeks to make one's children (or someone else's children) after one's own image (or an image of one's choosing) and their future according to one's will. In some cases the despotism may be mild and benevolent. In other cases it will be mischievous and downright tyrannical. But despotism—the control of another through one's will—it inevitably will be.

Meeting Some Objections

The defenders of cloning, of course, are not wittingly friends of despotism. Indeed, they regard themselves mainly as friends of freedom: the freedom of individuals to reproduce, the freedom of scientists and inventors to discover and devise and to foster "progress" in genetic knowledge and technique. They want large-scale cloning only for animals, but they wish to preserve cloning as a human option for exercising our "right to reproduce"—our right to have children, and children with "desirable genes." As law professor John Robertson points out, under our "right to reproduce" we already practice early forms of unnatural, artificial, and extramarital reproduction, and we already practice early forms of eugenic choice. For that reason, he argues, cloning is no big deal.

We have here a perfect example of the logic of the slippery slope, and the slippery way in which it already works in that area. Only a few years ago, slippery-slope arguments were advanced to oppose artificial insemination and in vitro fertilization using unrelated sperm donors. Principles used to justify those practices, it was said, will be used to justify more artificial and more eugenic practices, including cloning. Not so, the defenders retorted, since we can make the necessary distinctions. And now, without even a gesture at making the necessary distinctions, the continuity of practice is held by itself to be justificatory.

The principle of reproductive freedom as currently enunciated by the proponents of cloning logically embraces the ethical acceptability of sliding down the entire rest of the slope—to producing children ectogenetically from sperm to term (should it become feasible) and to producing children whose entire genetic makeup will be the product of parental eugenic planning and choice. If reproductive freedom means the right to have a child of one's own choosing, by whatever means, it knows and accepts no limits.

But, far from being legitimated by a "right to reproduce," the emergence of techniques of assisted reproduction and genetic engineering should compel us to reconsider the meaning and limits of such a putative right. In truth, a "right to reproduce" has always been a peculiar and problematic notion. Rights generally belong to individuals, but this is a right that (before cloning) no one can exercise alone. Does the right then inhere only in couples? Only in married couples? Is it a (woman's) right to carry or deliver or a right (of one or more parents) to nurture and rear? Is it a right to have your own biological child? Is it a right only to attempt reproduction or a right also to succeed? Is it a right to acquire the baby of one's choice?

The assertion of a negative "right to reproduce" certainly makes sense when it claims protection against state interference with procreative liberty, say, through a program of compulsory sterilization. But surely it cannot be the basis of a tort claim against nature, to be made good by technology, should free efforts at natural procreation fail. Some insist that the right to reproduce embraces also the right against state interference with the free use of all technological means to obtain a child. Yet such a position can-

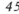

not be sustained: for reasons having to do with the means employed, any community may rightfully prohibit surrogate pregnancy, polygamy, or the sale of babies to infertile couples without violating anyone's basic human "right to reproduce." When the exercise of a previously innocuous freedom now involves or impinges on troublesome practices that the original freedom never was intended to reach, the general presumption of liberty needs to be reconsidered.

We do indeed already practice negative eugenic selection, through genetic screening and prenatal diagnosis. Yet our practices are governed by a norm of health. We seek to prevent the birth of children who suffer from known (serious) genetic diseases. When and if gene therapy becomes possible, such diseases could then be treated, in utero or even before implantation. I have no ethical objection in principle to such a practice (though I have some practical worries), precisely because it serves the medical goal of healing existing individuals. But therapy, to be therapy, implies not only an existing "patient." It also implies a norm of health. In this respect, even germline gene "therapy," though practiced not on a human being but on egg and sperm, is less radical than cloning, which is in no way therapeutic. But once one blurs the distinction between health promotion and genetic enhancement, between so-called negative and positive eugenics, one opens the door to all future eugenic designs. "To make sure that a child will be healthy and have good chances in life": that is Robertson's principle, and, owing to its latter clause, it is an utterly elastic principle, with no boundaries. Being over eight feet tall will likely produce some very good chances in life, and so will having the looks of Marilyn Monroe, and so will a genius-level intelligence.

Proponents want us to believe that there are legitimate uses of cloning that can be distinguished from illegitimate uses, but by their own principles no such limits can be found. (Nor could any such limits be enforced in practice.) Reproductive freedom, as they understand it, is governed solely by the subjective wishes of the parents-to-be (plus the avoidance of bodily harm to the child). The sentimentally appealing case of the childless married couple is, on those grounds, indistinguishable from the case of an individual (married or not) who would like to clone someone famous or talented, living or dead. Further, the principle here endorsed justifies not only cloning but, indeed, all future artificial attempts to create (manufacture) "perfect" babies.

A concrete example will show how, in practice no less than in principle, the so-called innocent case will merge with, or even turn into, the more troubling ones. In practice, the eager parent-to-be will necessarily be subject to the tyranny of expertise. Consider an infertile married couple, she lacking eggs or he lacking sperm, that wants a child of their (genetic) own and proposes to clone either husband or wife. The scientist-physician (who is also coowner of the cloning company) points out the likely difficulties: A cloned child is not really their (genetic) child, but the child of only *one* of them; that imbalance may produce strains on the marriage; the child might suffer identity confusion; there is a risk of perpetuating the cause of sterility. The scientist-physician also points out the advantages of choosing a donor nucleus. Far better than a child of their own would be a child of their own choosing. Touting his own expertise in selecting healthy and talented donors, the doctor presents the couple with his latest catalog containing the pictures, the health records, and the accomplishments of his stable of cloning donors, samples of whose tissues are in his deep freeze. Why not, dearly beloved, a more perfect baby?

The "perfect baby," of course, is the project not of the

infertility doctors, but of the eugenic scientists and their supporters. For them, the paramount right is not the so-called right to reproduce but what biologist Bentley Glass called, a quarter of a century ago, "the right of every child to be born with a sound physical and mental constitution, based on a sound genotype . . . the inalienable right to a sound heritage." But to secure that right and to achieve the requisite quality control over new human life, human conception and gestation will need to be brought fully into the bright light of the laboratory, beneath which the child-to-be can be fertilized, nourished, pruned, weeded, watched, inspected, prodded, pinched, cajoled, injected, tested, rated, graded, approved, stamped, wrapped, sealed, and delivered. There is no other way to produce the perfect baby.

Yet we are urged by proponents of cloning to forget about the science fiction scenarios of laboratory manufacture and multiple-copied clones and to focus only on the homely cases of infertile couples exercising their reproductive rights. But why, if the single cases are so innocent, should multiplying their performance be so off-putting? (Similarly, why do others object to people's making money from that practice if the practice itself is perfectly acceptable?) When we follow the sound ethical principle of universalizing our choice—would it be right if everyone cloned a Wilt Chamberlain (with his consent, of course)? would it be right if everyone decided to practice asexual reproduction?—we discover what is wrong with such seemingly innocent cases. The so-called science fiction cases make vivid the meaning of what looks to us, mistakenly, to be benign.

Though I recognize certain continuities between cloning and, say, in vitro fertilization, I believe that cloning differs in essential and important ways. Yet those who disagree should be reminded that the "continuity" argument cuts both ways. Sometimes we establish bad precedents and discover that they were bad only when we follow their inexorable logic to places we never meant to go. Can the defenders of cloning show us today how, on their principles, we shall be able to see producing babies ("perfect babies") entirely in the laboratory or exercising full control over their genotypes (including so-called enhancement) as ethically different, in any essential way, from present forms of assisted reproduction? Or are they willing to admit, despite their attachment to the principle of continuity, that the complete obliteration of "mother" or "father," the complete depersonalization of procreation, the complete manufacture of human beings, and the complete genetic control of one generation over the next would be ethically problematic and essentially different from current forms of assisted reproduction? If so, where and how will they draw the line, and why? I draw it at cloning, for all the reasons given.

Ban the Cloning of Humans

What, then, should we do? We should declare that human cloning is unethical in itself and dangerous in its likely consequences. In so doing, we shall have the backing of the overwhelming majority of our fellow Americans, of the human race, and (I believe) of most practicing scientists. Next, we should do all that we can to prevent the cloning of human beings. We should do that by means of an international legal ban if possible and by a unilateral national ban at a minimum. Scientists may secretly undertake to violate such a law, but they will be deterred by not being able to stand up proudly to claim the credit for their technological bravado and success. Such a ban on clonal babymaking, moreover, will not harm the progress of basic genetic science and technology. On the contrary, it will reassure the public that scientists are happy to proceed without violating the deep ethical norms and intuitions of the human community.

That still leaves the vexed question about laboratory research using early embryonic human clones, specially created only for such research purposes, with no intention to implant them into a uterus. There is no question that such research holds great promise for gaining fundamental knowledge about normal (and abnormal) differentiation and for developing tissue lines for transplantation that might be used, say, in treating leukemia or in repairing brain or spinal cord injuries—to mention just a few of the conceivable benefits. Still, unrestricted clonal embryo research will surely make the production of living human clones much more likely. Once the genies put the cloned embryos into the bottles, who can strictly control where they go, especially in the absence of legal prohibitions against implanting them to produce a child?

I appreciate the potentially great gains in scientific knowledge and medical treatment available from embryo research, especially with cloned embryos. At the same time, I have serious reservations about creating human embryos for the sole purpose of experimentation. There is something deeply repugnant and fundamentally transgressive about such a utilitarian treatment of prospective human life. Such total, shameless exploitation is worse, in my opinion, than the "mere" destruction of nascent life. But I see no added objections, as a matter of principle, to creating and using *cloned* early embryos for research purposes, beyond the objections that I might raise to doing so with embryos produced sexually.

And yet, as a matter of policy and prudence, any opponent of the manufacture of cloned humans must, I think, in the end oppose also the creating of cloned human embryos. Frozen embryonic clones (belonging to whom?) can be shuttled around without detection. Commercial ventures in human cloning will be developed without adequate oversight. To build a fence around the law, prudence dictates that one oppose—for that reason alone—all production of cloned human embryos, even for research purposes. We should allow all cloning research on animals to go forward, but the only defensible barrier we can erect against the slippery slide, I suspect, is to insist on the inviolable distinction between animal and human cloning.

Some readers and certainly most scientists will not accept such prudent restraints, since they desire the benefits of research. They will prefer, even in fear and trembling, to allow human embryo cloning research to go forward.

Very well. Let us test them. If the scientists want to be taken seriously on ethical grounds, they must at the very least agree that embryonic research may proceed if and only if it is preceded by an absolute and effective ban on all attempts to implant into a uterus a cloned human embryo (cloned from an adult) to produce a living child. Absolutely no permission for the former without the latter.

The National Bioethics Advisory Commission's recommendations regarding these matters were a step in the right direction, but a step made limpingly and without adequate support. To its credit, the commission has indeed called for federal legislation to prevent anyone from attempting to create a child through cloning. That was, frankly, more than I expected. But the *moral basis* for the commission's opposition to cloning is, sadly, much less than expected and needed, and the ban it urges is to be only temporary. Trying to clone a human being, says the commission, is "morally unacceptable" "*at this time*" because the technique has not been perfected to the point of safe usage. In other words, once it becomes readily feasible to clone a human being, with little risk of bodily harm to the resulting child, the commission has offered not one agreed-upon reason to object. Indeed, anticipating such improvements in technique, the commission insists that "it is critical" that any legislative ban on baby-making through cloning "should include a sunset clause to ensure that Congress will review the issue after a specified time period (three to five years) to decide whether the prohibition continues to be needed." Although it identifies other ethical concerns (beyond the issue of safety), that blue-ribbon ethics commission takes no stand on any of them! It says only that those issues "require much more widespread and careful public deliberation *before this technology may be used*"—not to decide *whether* the technology *should* be used. Relativistically, the commission wants to ensure only that such ethical and social issues be regularly reviewed "in light of public understandings at that time." This is hardly the sort of opposition to cloning that could be made the basis of any lasting prohibition.

Almost as worrisome, the report is silent on the vexed question of creating cloned human embryos for use in research. Silence is, of course, not an endorsement, but neither is it opposition. Given the currently existing ban on the use of federal funds for any research that involves cre-

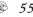

ating human embryos for experimentation, the commission may have preferred to avoid needless controversy by addressing that issue. Besides, those commissioners (no doubt a big majority) who favor proceeding with cloned embryo research have in fact gained their goal precisely by silence: both the moratorium on federal funding and the legislative ban called for by the commission are confined *solely* to attempts to *create a child* through cloning. The commission knows well how vigorously and rapidly embryo research is progressing in the private sector, and the commission surely understands that its silence on the subject—along with Congress's—means that the creation of human embryonic clones will proceed and perhaps is already proceeding in private or commercial laboratories. Indeed, the report expects and tacitly welcomes such human embryo research: for by what other means shall we arrive at the expected improvements in human cloning technology that would require the recommended periodic reconsideration of any legislative ban?

In the end, the report of the commission turns out to be a moral and (despite its best efforts) a practical failure. Morally, this ethics commission has waffled on the main ethical question by refusing to declare the production of human clones unethical (or ethical). Practically, the moratorium and ban on baby-making that it calls for, while welcome as temporary restraints, have not been given the justification needed to provide a solid and lasting protection against the production of cloned human beings. To the contrary, the commission's weak ethical stance may be said to undermine even its limited call for restraint. Do we really need a federal law solely to protect unborn babies from bodily harm?

Opponents of cloning need therefore to be vigilant. They should press for legislation to *permanently* prohibit baby-making through cloning, and they should take steps to make such a prohibition effective.

The proposal for such a legislative ban is without American precedent, at least in technological matters, though the British and others have banned cloning of human beings, and we ourselves ban incest, polygamy, and other forms of "reproductive freedom." Needless to say, working out the details of such a ban, especially a global one, would be tricky, what with the need to develop appropriate sanctions for violators. Perhaps such a ban will prove ineffective; perhaps it will eventually be shown to have been a mistake. But it would at least place the burden of practical proof where it belongs: on the proponents of this horror, requiring them to show very clearly what great social or medical good can be had only by the cloning of human beings.

We Americans have lived by, and prospered under, a rosy optimism about scientific and technological progress. The technological imperative—if it can be done, it must be done—has probably served us well, though we should admit that there is no accurate method for weighing benefits and harms. Even when, as in the cases of environmental pollution, urban decay, or the lingering deaths that are the unintended byproducts of medical success, we recognize the unwelcome outcomes of technological advance, we remain confident in our ability to fix all the "bad" consequences—usually by means of still newer and better technologies. How successful we can continue to be in such post hoc repairing is at least an open question. But there is very good reason for shifting the paradigm around, at least regarding those technological interventions into the human body and mind that will surely effect fundamental (and likely irreversible) changes in human nature, basic human relationships, and what it means to be a human being. Here we surely should not be willing to risk everything in the naïve hope that, should things go wrong, we can later set them right.

The president's call for a moratorium on human cloning has given us an important opportunity. In a truly unprecedented way, we can strike a blow for the human control of the technological project, for wisdom, prudence, and human dignity. The prospect of human cloning, so repulsive to contemplate, is the occasion for deciding whether we shall be slaves of unregulated progress, and ultimately its artifacts, or whether we shall remain free human beings who guide our technique toward the enhancement of human dignity. If we are to seize the occasion, we must, as the late Paul Ramsey wrote,

> raise the ethical questions with a serious and not a frivolous conscience. A man of frivolous conscience announces that there are ethical quandaries ahead that we must urgently consider before the future catches up with us. By this he often means that we need to devise a new ethics that will provide the rationalization for doing in the future what men are bound to do because of new actions and interventions science will have made possible. In contrast a man

of serious conscience means to say in raising urgent ethical questions that there may be some things that men should never do. The good things that men do can be made complete only by the things they refuse to do.

The Paradox of Cloning

James Q. Wilson

*L*et us suppose that it becomes possible to clone human beings. The creation of Dolly the cloned sheep makes this more likely than anyone once suspected. How should we react to that event?

Like most people, I instinctively recoil from the idea. There is, I think, a natural sentiment that is offended by the mental picture of identical babies being produced in some biological factory. When we hear a beautiful model say that she would like to have a clone of herself, we are puzzled. When we recall *The Boys from Brazil*, a story of identical offspring of Adolf Hitler being raised to further his horrible work, we are outraged.

But before deciding what we think about cloning, we ought to pause and identify more precisely what it is about the process that is so distressing. My preliminary view is that the central problem is not creating an identical twin but creating it without parents.

Happily, we need not react immediately to human cloning. The task of moving from one sheep to many sheep, and from sheep to other animals, and from animals to humans will be long and difficult. Dolly was the only lamb to emerge out of 277 attempts, and we still do not know how long she will live or what diseases, if any, she might contract.

And the risks attendant on a hasty reaction are great. A premature ban on any scientific effort moving in the direction of cloning could well impede useful research on the genetic basis of diseases or on opportunities for improving agriculture. Already a great deal of work is underway on modifying the genetic structure of laboratory animals to study illnesses and to generate human proteins and antibodies. Aware of the value of genetic research, several members of Congress have expressed reservations about quick legislative action. Nevertheless, bills to ban cloning research have been introduced.

But even if such bills pass, the argument will be far from over. Congress may regulate or even block cloning research in the United States, but other countries are free to pursue their own strategies. If cloning is illegal in America but legal in Japan or China, Americans will go to those countries as cloning techniques are perfected. Science cannot be stopped. We should have learned that from the way we regulate drug treatments. We can ban a risky but useful drug, but the only effect is to limit its use to those who are willing and able to pay the airfare to Hong Kong.

Philosophical and Utilitarian Objections to Cloning

There are both philosophical and utilitarian objections to cloning. Two philosophical objections exist. The first is that cloning violates God's will by creating an infant in a way that does not depend on human sexual congress or make possible the divine inculcation of a soul. That is true, but so does in vitro fertilization. An egg and a sperm are united outside the human body in a glass container. The fertilized egg is then put into the body of either the woman who produced it or another woman hired to bear the infant. When first proposed, in vitro fertilization was ethically suspect. Today, it is generally accepted—and for good reason. Science supplies what one or both human bodies lack, namely, a reasonable chance to produce an infant. Surely God can endow that infant with a soul. Cloning, of course, removes one of the conjugal partners, but it is hard to imagine that God's desire to bestow a unique soul can be blocked by the fact that the infant does not result from an egg and sperm's joining but instead arises from an embryonic egg's reproducing itself.

The other philosophical objection is that cloning is contrary to nature. That is often asserted by critics of cloning who do not believe in an active God. I sympathize with that reaction, but few critics have yet made clear to me what compelling aspect of nature cloning violates. To the extent that such an objection has meaning, I think it must arise from the danger that the cloned child will be put to various harmful uses. If so, the objection cannot easily be distinguished from the more practical problems.

One set of those problems requires us to imagine scientists' cloning children to harvest organs and body parts or to produce for later use many Adolf Hitlers or Saddam Husseins. I have no doubt that there will arise mad scientists willing to do those things. After all, they have already created poison gas and conducted grisly experiments on prisoners of war and concentration-camp inmates.

The Importance of Parental Ties

But under what circumstances will such abuses occur? Largely, I think, when the cloned child has no parents. Parents, whether they acquire a child by normal birth, artificial insemination, or adoption, will, in the overwhelming majority of cases, become deeply attached to the infant and care for it without regard to its origin. The parental tie is not infallible—infanticide occurs, and some neonates are abandoned in trash bins—but it is powerful and largely independent of the origin of the child. If cloning is to occur, the central problem is to ensure that it be done only for two-parent families who want a child for their own benefit. We should remember that a clone must be borne by a female; it cannot be given birth in a laboratory. A human mother will carry a human clone; she and her husband will determine its fate. Hardly any parents, I think, would allow their child to be used as an organ bank for defective adults or as the next-generation proxy for a malevolent dictator. If the cloned child is born in the same way as a child resulting from marital congress, can it matter to the parents how it was conceived? And if it does not matter to the parents, should it matter to us?

We already have a kind of clone: identical twins. They are genetically identical humans. I have not heard of any twin's being used against its will as an unwitting organ bank for its brother or sister. Some may surrender a kidney or bone marrow to their sibling; many may give blood; but none, I think, has been "harvested." The idea that a cloned infant, born to its mother, would be treated differently is, I think, quite far-fetched.

At some time in the future, science may discover a way to produce a clone entirely in the laboratory. That we should ban. Without human birth, the parents' attitude toward the infant will be deeply compromised. Getting a clone from a laboratory would be like getting a puppy from a pet store: Both creatures might be charming, but neither would belong in any meaningful emotional sense to the owner. And unclaimed clones would be disposed of the same way as unclaimed puppies—killed.

There may be parents who, out of fear or ideology, can be persuaded to accept a clone of a Hussein in hopes that they can help produce an unending chain of vicious leaders. That is less far-fetched. We already know from the study of identical twins reared in different families that they are remarkably similar. A cloned Hussein would have an IQ close to that of his father and a personality that (insofar as we can measure such things) would have roughly a 50 percent chance of being like his. Each clone would be like an identical twin: nearly the same in appearance, very similar in intelligence and manner, and alike (but not a duplicate) in personality. We know that the environment will have some effect on each twin's personality, but it is easy to overestimate that. I am struck by how many scientists interested in cloning have reflexively adopted the view that the environment will have a powerful effect on a cloned child. (Cloning seems to have given a large boost to environmentalists.) But that reaction is exaggerated. From the work of Dr. Thomas Bouchard at the University of Minnesota, we know that giving identical twins different environments produces only slightly greater differences in character.

Our best hope for guarding against the duplication of a Saddam Hussein is a practical one. Any cloned offspring would reach maturity forty or so years after his father was born, and by then so much would have changed—Hussein, Sr., would probably not even be in power, and his country's political system might have been profoundly altered—that it is unlikely that Hussein, Jr., could do what his father did.

We do not know how many parents will request cloning, but some will. Suppose that the father cannot provide sperm or the mother is unable to produce a fertilizable egg. Such a family now has only three choices—remain childless, adopt, or arrange some form of assisted reproduction involving the sperm, egg, or even womb of a third party (artificial insemination, in vitro fertilization, or surrogate motherhood). Cloning would create a fourth choice: duplicate the father or the mother. Some parents who do not want to remain childless will find the last choice more attractive than adoption, which introduces a wholly new and largely unknown genetic factor into their family tree. Cloning guarantees that the child's genetic makeup will be identical to that of whichever parent is cloned.

Diversity for the Welfare of the Species

There is, of course, a risk that cloning may increase the number of surrogate mothers, with all the heartbreak and legal complexities that that entails, but I suspect that surrogates would be no more common for clones than they are for babies conceived in vitro.

More troubling is the possibility that a lesbian couple will use cloning to produce a child. Do we wish to make it easy for a homosexual pair to have children? Governments have different policies on that; let me set aside discussion of that matter for another occasion.

There is one important practical objection to the widespread use of cloning. As every evolutionary scientist knows, the survival of a species depends on two forces—environmental change that rewards some creatures and penalizes others and sufficient diversity among the species that, no matter what the environment, some members of the species will benefit.

Cloning creates the opportunity for people to maximize a valued trait. Suppose we wish to have children with a high IQ, an athletic physique, easily tanned skin, or freedom from a particular genetic disease. By cloning persons who have the desired trait, we can guarantee that the trait will appear in the infant.

That may make good sense to parents, but it is bad news for the species. We have no way of knowing what environmental challenges will confront us in the future. Traits that today are desirable may become irrelevant or harmful in the future; traits that now are unappealing may become essential for human survival in the centuries ahead.

That problem is one for which there is no obvious individual solution. People maximizing the welfare of their infant can inhibit the welfare of the species. One way to constrain a couple's efforts to secure the "perfect" child would be to restrict their choice of genes to either the father or the mother. They could secure a specific genetic product, but they could not obtain what they might think is the ideal product.

But the real constraint on the misuse of cloning comes from a simple human tendency. Many parents do not want a child with particular traits. Conception is a lottery. It produces an offspring that gets roughly half its genes from its father and half from its mother, but the mixture occurs in unpredictable and fascinating combinations. All parents spend countless delightful hours wondering whether the child has its mother's eyes or its father's smile or its grandfather's nose or its grandmother's personality. And they watch in wonder as the infant becomes an adult with its own unique personality and mannerisms.

I think that most people prefer the lottery to certainty. (I know they prefer sex to cloning.) Lured by the lottery, they help meet the species' need for biological diversity. Moreover, if parents are tempted by certainty but limited to cells taken from either the father or the mother, they will have to ask themselves hard questions.

Do I want another man like the father, who is smart and earns a lot—but whose hair is receding, who has diabetes, and who is so obsessed with work that he is not much fun on weekends? Or do I want another woman like the mother, who is bright and sweet—but who has bad teeth, a family risk of breast cancer, and sleeps too late in the morning?

Not many of us know perfect people, least of all our own parents. If we want to clone a person, most of us will think twice about cloning somebody we already know well. And if we can clone only from among our own family, our desire to do it at all will be much weakened. Perhaps parents' love of entering the reproductive lottery is itself a revelation of evolution at work, one designed to help maintain biological diversity.

In one special case we may want to clone a creature well known to us. My friend Heather Higgins has said that cloning our pets—or at least some pets—may make sense. I would love to have another Labrador retriever just like Winston and another pair of cats exactly like Sarah and Clementine.

Ethical Human Cloning

The central question facing those who approach cloning with an open mind is whether the gains from human cloning—a remedy for infertility and substitute for adoption—are worth the risks of farming organs, propagating dictators, and impeding evolution. I think that, provided certain conditions are met, the gains will turn out to exceed the risks.

The conditions are those to which I have already referred. Cloning should be permitted only on behalf of two married partners, and the mother should—absent some special medical condition that doctors must certify—carry the fertile tissue to birth. Then the offspring would belong to the parents. That parental constraint would prevent organ farming and the indiscriminate or political misuse of cloning technology.

The major threat cloning produces is a further weakening of the two-parent family. Cloning humans, if it can occur at all, cannot be prevented, but cloning unmarried persons will expand the greatest cultural problem our country now faces. A cloned child, so far as we now know, cannot be produced in a laboratory. A mother must give it birth. Dolly had a mother, and if humans are produced the same way, they will have mothers, also. But not, I hope, unmarried mothers. Indeed, given the likely expense and difficulty of cloning, and the absence from it of any sexual pleasure, we are unlikely to see many unmarried teenage girls choosing that method. If unmarried cloning occurs, it is likely to be among affluent persons who think that they are entitled to act without the restraints and burdens of family life. They are wrong.

Of course, an unmarried or unscrupulous person eager for a cloned offspring may travel from the United States to a place where there are no restrictions of the sort I suggest. There is no way to prevent that. We can try to curtail it by telling anyone who returns to this country with a child born abroad to an American citizen that one of two conditions must be met before the child will be regarded as an American citizen. The parent bringing it back must show by competent medical evidence either that the child is the product of a normal (noncloned) birth or adoption or that the child, though the product of cloning, belongs to a married couple who will be responsible for it. Failing that, the child could not become an American citizen. But, of course, some people would evade any restrictions. There is, in short, no way that American law can produce a fail-safe restraint on undesirable cloning.

My view—that cloning presents no special ethical risks if society does all in its power to establish that the child is born to a married woman and is the joint responsibility of the married couple—will not satisfy those whose objections to cloning are chiefly religious. If man is made in the image of God, can man make himself (by cloning) and still be in God's image? I would suggest that producing a fertilized egg by sexual contact does not uniquely determine that image and therefore that nonsexual, in vitro fertilization is acceptable. And if that is so, then nonsexually transplanting cell nuclei into enucleated eggs might also be acceptable.

That is not a view that will commend itself to many devout Christians or Jews. I would ask of them only that they explain what it is about sexual fertilization that so affects God's judgment about the child that results.

Part Two

Family Needs Its Natural Roots

Leon R. Kass

$\mathcal{N}$o reasonable person should ever feel comfortable finding himself in disagreement with James Q. Wilson, always the voice of sanity and a bastion of practical wisdom. Discovering myself in such an unenviable position, I have studied his essay with some care, partly to allow his arguments to work on me, partly to discover why we have reached such different conclusions. Though I would prefer to share his reassuring outlook, I remain unpersuaded of the ethical innocence of cloning and perplexed about why the usually sage Professor Wilson seems this time to be playing Dr. Pangloss.

First, however, some points of agreement. Like Professor Wilson, I am not especially worried about possible political abuses of cloning, for example, the mass production of identical clones or the replication of dictators, or about threats to human evolution. I also agree that, at least in the short run, cloning is unlikely to be widely used as a means of satisfying the reproductive desires of married couples. Professor Wilson and I share a deep commitment to marriage and the normal two-parent family, primarily because we care about the well-being of children. And I am willing to concede that a cloned child, if born of woman and *if* cared for lovingly and responsibly within a marriage *like any other child* (a big if), could turn out to be no worse or less happy a person than he or I—that would be an empirical question, not resolvable as a matter of principle. But I cannot share Professor Wilson's optimism that the practice can be confined to such seemingly innocent intramarital cases. Moreover, I do not find even those cases to be innocent. On the contrary, for the specific reasons I have elaborated in my essay, I regard cloning to be *in itself* a form of child abuse, even if no one complains, and a deep violation of our given nature as gendered and engendering beings.

Accommodating Utilitarians

Professor Wilson begins, as I do, with repugnance. He acknowledges his own "instinctive recoil" from the idea of human cloning. But, surprisingly for someone who has al-

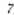

most single-handedly restored our awareness of the importance of a prearticulate human moral sense and who ultimately relies on that sense to save us from the abuses of cloning, he does not quite trust his own sense of moral disquiet and sets out to explain it with reasons. Whether he intends it or not, that move places the burden of proof on those who object to cloning rather than on the proponents. Worse, it requires that the reasons offered be finally acceptable to utilitarians who measure only in terms of tangible harms and benefits but who are generally blind to the deeper meanings of things.

Before settling into his own utilitarian arguments, Professor Wilson nods in the direction of philosophical and religious objections, but his treatment of those is superficial. No thoughtful theologian objects to assisted reproduction because it limits God's power to inculcate a human soul; theologians worry not about the impotence of God but about the hubris of man. In addition, they have a great deal to say about the meaning of human procreation and its relation to the sacrament of marriage. (Though they speak not from my own tradition, there is much anyone can learn from Anglican Oliver O'Donovan's *Begotten or Made?,* Methodist Paul Ramsey's *Fabricated Man,* and the Roman Catholic Congregation for the Doctrine of the

Faith's Instruction on "The Dignity of Procreation.") Moreover, Professor Wilson's use of the *social* acceptance of in vitro fertilization—at first "ethically suspect," today "generally accepted, and for good reason"—to rebut religious objections against laboratory conception of human life cannot be taken seriously: Does the growing social acceptability of sodomy or adultery constitute a refutation of Leviticus 18:22 or the Seventh Commandment?

The Moral Pointings of Nature

By removing human conception from the human body and by introducing new partners in reproduction (scientists and physicians), in vitro fertilization did more than "supply what one or both bodies lack, namely, a reasonable chance to produce an infant." By putting the origin of human life literally in human hands, it began a process that would lead, in practice, to the increasing technical mastery of human generation and, in thought, to the continuing erosion of respect for the mystery of sexuality and human renewal. The very existence of in vitro fertilization, notwithstanding its real benefits, also becomes a justification for the next steps in turning procreation into manufacture (Professor Wilson is already singing the song of that slippery slope), not least because it obscures the deeper meaning of the naturally significant relations among embodiment, sexual differentiation, and procreation. The arrival of cloning, far from gaining legitimacy from the precedent of in vitro fertilization, should rather awaken those who previously saw no difficulty with starting human life in petri dishes.

Professor Wilson does profess sympathy with those who think cloning is contrary to nature, but—thanks largely to the veil technology has dropped over nature and to modern science's earlier dismissal of natural teleology—nature in its possibly normative pointings has become invisible to him. To him (and to many others), but not to me. Here is probably the biggest philosophical reason for our difference.

One way to put that difference is to claim, as Christopher DeMuth commented to me, that Professor Wilson thinks that the issue is marriage and family whereas I think that the issue is sex. At first glance that observation is sound enough: At the center of my argument is a discussion of the "profundity of sex"; at the center of Professor Wilson's is the concern that all children have parents. But the difference is more apparent than real, especially if one understands the generative meaning of sexuality and, even more, if one sees—as Professor Wilson perhaps does not—that one will be increasingly incapable of defending the institution of marriage and the two-parent family if one is indifferent to its natural grounding in what I call the ontology of sex. Can we ensure, even in thought, that all children will have two parents if we ignore, in our social arrangements, the *natural* (hetero)*sexual* ground of parenthood?

I began with sexuality, first of all, because cloning is *a*sexual reproduction. Generatively speaking, the essence of sexuality is not the concourse of bodies in coitus (fish, for example, practice sexual reproduction, but the eggs are fertilized outside the body), but rather the biparental (male and female) contributions to new life. (In vitro fertilization is thus, in that profound sense, *sexual* reproduction, albeit not very sexy.) A clone, because asexually reproduced, lacks two parents; though I have called it a single-parent child, it would be more accurate to say that, since it is the twin rather than the offspring of its "source," it has *no* parents, biologically speaking—unless its "parents" are the mother and father of the person from whom it was cloned.

Professor Wilson, not without reason, looks away from the sources of the conceptus and is willing to define motherhood solely by the act of giving birth. And if the clone's birth mother is married, her husband will be, by (social) definition, its father—as he agrees to be, by marrying her, of all children she may bear (regardless of biological paternity). In that way Professor Wilson tries to give a virtually normal social biparental identity to this radically aparental child, clinging himself, in doing so, to nature and the (still) natural facts of gestation and parturition as his anchor. (For that reason he would ban ectogenesis, the laboratory growth of a "newborn" child from sperm to term: "Without human birth, the parents' attitude toward the infant would be deeply compromised"; opponents can easily point out, however, that parents who adopt children are able to love them without regard to where they came from.) But that view runs into difficulty with surrogate mothers, who could be said to be, like the scientists, just supplying to a wombless woman and her husband a reasonable chance of a child of their own. More important for the case of cloning, Professor Wilson ignores the fact that giving birth to one's twin sister does not exactly reproduce a normal mother-daughter relationship.

The Evils of Intrafamilial Cloning

By playing down the psychological issue of identity and individuality, Professor Wilson is able to treat as innocent the prospect of intrafamilial cloning—cloning of husband or wife. But even the defenders of cloning readily acknowledge the unique dangers of mixing the twin relation with the parent-child relation. (For that situation, the relation of contemporaneous identical twins is no precedent; yet even this less problematic case teaches us how difficult it is to wrest independence from the being with whom one has the most powerful affinity.) Virtually no parent is going to be able to treat a clone of himself or herself as one does a child generated by the lottery of sex. The new life will constantly be scrutinized in relation to that of the older copy. Even in the absence of unusual parental expectations for the clone—say, to live the same life, only without its errors—the child is likely to be ever a curiosity, ever a potential source of *déjà vu*. Moreover, clones, because they are the flesh and blood (and the look-alike) of only one parent, are likely to be especially implicated in tensions between the parents. In the event of a divorce, will mommy still love the clone of daddy? One might almost dare assert that any couple incapable of seeing in advance the dangers of intrafamilial cloning shows itself unfit for parenting such a child.

Reproductive Freedom and Technology Undermine Family and Parenthood

Professor Wilson is also naïve in believing that cloning can be confined to married couples seeking merely a remedy

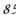

for childlessness. In vitro fertilization has not been so restricted; single women now use artificial insemination with donor sperm, both in vivo and in vitro. Commercial sperm banks are apparently thriving, including some that specialize in eugenic germinal choice (sperm from geniuses). Couples interested in cloning, especially those who have figured out the dangers of self-cloning, will certainly want to make use of "high-class" donor nuclei. (But notice that for people willing to go outside the marriage for sources of gametes, in vitro fertilization with donor sperm and embryo donation are already alternatives to cloning, so there is almost no one for whom cloning is the only alternative to either childlessness or adoption.) Cloning provides the powerful opening salvo in the campaign to exercise control over the quality of offspring.

Given our current beliefs about reproductive freedom, the fracture of the once-respected and solid bonds among sex, love, procreation, and stable marriage, and the relentless march of technology, it will prove impossible to preserve Professor Wilson's faint hopes for family and parenthood—in the absence of some miraculous recovery of good sense about sexuality and the meaning of procreation and an attitude that once again sees children as a gift to be treasured rather than as a product for our manipulation. The right to reproduce (or not) is now widely regarded as a right belonging to individuals: Who are Professor Wilson and I to stand in the way of any woman's desire for personal self-fulfillment through motherhood? (The legal battle concerning the true locus of reproductive rights was lost in the 1960s over contraception: A husband and wife's right of *marital* privacy that overthrew laws barring the sale of contraceptives to married couples—*Griswold* v. *Connecticut*—almost immediately became an *individual's* right of *sexual* privacy, married or not—*Eisenstadt* v. *Baird*.) The meaning of the right to reproduce is also being expanded to include a right to the child of one's choice. Parents already exercise some choice, through genetic screening, over the quality of their children—and this even with science's ability to alter genotype still in its infancy. Strange requests are already being voiced. Lobbyists for the congenitally deaf are seeking to abort the nonimpaired fetuses as part of their campaign to "normalize" deafness and to provide only deaf children for the deaf. Gay-rights organizations urged the National Bioethics Advisory Commission to declare in favor of cloning; some even argued that, should homosexuality be shown to have a genetic basis, homosexuals would have an obligation to reproduce through cloning to preserve their kind! Given the state of our culture, it is rather late in the sexual day for Professor Wilson's call to rally the family wagons to protect the little beloved clone.

Professor Wilson is surely right to worry about the risks of legislative prohibitions of scientific practices—though he would himself seem to need legislation to keep cloning within the family. And he is right again in recognizing that such legislation is neither foolproof nor immune to circumvention by travel to more permissive localities (though I am confident that he would not for those reasons urge us to repeal our laws against incest or polygamy, nor would he have us refrain from outlawing growing babies in bottles just because the technology were available or because the Chinese or someone else were doing it). Also, as a practical matter, he appears to be content to permit cloning so long as cloning remains a marginal practice. On that point I part company.

A Shudderless Society

Even if human cloning is rarely undertaken, a society in which it is tolerated is no longer the same society—any more than is a society that permits (even small-scale) incest or cannibalism or slavery. It is a society that has forgotten how to shudder, that always rationalizes away the abominable. A society that allows cloning has, whether it knows it or not, tacitly said yes to converting procreation into manufacture and to treating our children as pure projects of our will. Indeed, the principles here legitimated could—and will—be used to legitimate the entire humanitarian superhighway to *Brave New World*. Professor Wilson's sweet reasonableness of today will come back to haunt him, once he sees what he has unknowingly said yes to. Better he should trust his immediate moral sense.

Sex and Family

James Q. Wilson

*L*eon Kass has written a deeply learned, splendidly argued, and emotionally compelling essay on cloning. It has caused me to rethink some of my views and, if I understand him well enough, I may change them. But first I wish to be certain that I understand him.

The essential difference between his view and mine is, I think, that I link the meaning of children to the existence of the family and he links it to the power of sexuality. In my view children born of a woman, however the conception is produced, will have in the great majority of cases that special, logically irrational, but socially and morally vital affection that has sustained human life for millennia. If she is married to a man and they, like the great majority of married couples, invest energy, love, and commitment in the child, the child is likely to do well.

Dr. Kass's view may overlap mine, but it is somewhat

different in emphasis. He worries that creating babies without marital sex is the fundamental error. He is distressed
by the prospect of children being "made rather than begotten" because that will weaken the "soul-elevating power
of sexuality" that has been established "by nature." "By
nature, each child has two complementary biological progenitors . . . . [And so] the precise genetic constitution of
the resulting offspring is determined by a combination of
nature and chance, not by human design." We are profoundly threatened, he suggests, by "asexual reproduction"
that produces "'single-parent' offspring." Such offspring will
experience confusion over their identity, suffer from being produced as "artifacts," and become the victims of "despotism." Asexual reproduction, in his view, is an effort to
maintain "self-preservation"; sexual reproduction, by contrast, implies that we are perishable: "when we are sexually active we are voting with our genitalia for our own demise."

I certainly agree with him that neither sex nor families
are "cultural constructs" invented by people who are now
free, in the name of personal liberation or political ideology, to uninvent them. I am uncertain, however, about how
far his interest in natural sexuality takes him.

If Dr. Kass thinks that sexuality is more important than

families, then he would object to any form of assisted reproduction that does not involve parental coition. Many such forms now exist. Children are adopted by parents who did not give them birth. Artificial insemination produces children without sexual congress. Some forms of such insemination rely on sperm produced by a man other than the woman's husband, while other forms involve the artificial insemination of a surrogate mother who will relinquish the baby to a married couple. By in vitro fertilization, eggs and sperm can be joined in a petri dish and then transferred into the woman's uterus.

I am not clear how Dr. Kass feels about those other methods of producing children. He alludes to the controversy that once surrounded those methods and acknowledges the fact that today tens of thousands of people now sustain over 200 assisted-reproduction clinics in this country. He implies, I think, that he finds much, perhaps all, of that to be unsettling. Adding cloning to the list of assisted reproduction methods reveals, he writes, the "logic of the slippery slope."

I have mixed views about assisted reproduction. Some I endorse, others I worry about, still others I oppose. The two principles on which my views rest concern, first, the special relationship between infant and mother that is the product of childbirth, however conception was arranged, and, second, the great advantage to children that comes from growing up in an intact, two-parent family.

The Value of Parental Bonds

Some studies suggest that adopted children are more likely to wind up with emotional problems, but the best research in this country suggests that children adopted at a very early age do about as well as children raised by their birth parents. The Colorado Adoption Project, perhaps the best studied American case, involves children adopted within one month of their birth. It found that those children do about as well in the hands of adoptive parents who did not produce them as do children raised by their birth parents. While it may be true, as Dr. Kass writes, that birth parents do not "deliberately produce children for adoption," the early surrender of a child to an adoptive family—in the Colorado Adoption Project, in about four days—indicates that some mothers come quite close to doing just that. The harmful effects on the child are minimal or nonexistent.

Since artificial insemination first produced a live human birth in 1978, its use has grown. Artificial insemination is now responsible for perhaps 1 percent of all first-child births in the Western world. In 1987 the Office of Technology Assessment studied some 11,000 American doctors providing artificial insemination to roughly 172,000 women. The great majority of the beneficiaries were married women who were trying to cope with male infertility. Roughly half the women managed to be inseminated by sperm drawn from their husbands and the other half from sperm taken from unknown donors. (The donors turned out to be medical and other graduate students, doctors, and hospital workers.) When performing artificial insemination with sperm from an unknown donor, most doctors were willing to screen the sperm's donor to match the patient's preferences for race, ethnicity, eye color, height, weight, and body type.

In another survey of the United States and Canada done in 1992 by a medical group, some 38,000 efforts at assisted reproduction were examined, most of them involving in vitro fertilization. The great majority used the birth mother's own eggs, but some—about 1,800—used donated eggs, mostly from anonymous donors.

Obviously, assisted reproduction, whether by artificial insemination or in vitro fertilization, is now relatively common. In none of those cases is the child the result of mari-

tal sex. And in some cases—perhaps half of all artificial in-
seminations and 5 percent of all in vitro fertilizations—the
child is not genetically related to at least one parent.

There have been several efforts to study how well the
children fare. I am aware of none that shows in vitro fertilization to have had a harmful effect on the children's
mental or psychological status or their relationships with
parents. One study in the Netherlands found children conceived by in vitro fertilization in two-parent families to be
the object of *more* maternal involvement and pleasure than
were children of similar parents whose offspring had been
conceived without in vitro fertilization.

A similar study in England compared children conceived
by in vitro fertilization or by artificial insemination with
sperm from an unknown donor with children who were
sexually conceived and grew up in either birth or adoptive
families. By every measure of parenting, the children who
were the product of either an artificial fertilization or insemination by a donor did better than children who were
naturally conceived. The better parenting of children conceived by in vitro fertilization or by artificial insemination
with sperm from an unknown donor should not be surprising. Those parents had been struggling to have children; when a new technology made it possible for them to

do what they had long wanted, they were delighted, and that delight motivated them to be especially warm toward and supportive of their offspring.

Paul Ramsey, whom Dr. Kass quotes, would not like any of those arrangements, whatever the effect on children. As he wrote in 1970, for any third party—say, an egg or sperm donor—to be involved violates the marriage covenant. That is also the view of the Roman Catholic Church. My view is different: If the child is born of a woman who is part of a two-parent family and both parents work hard to raise it properly, and if the child's life is not harmed by the fact that it was adopted, conceived artificially or in a petri dish, or even conceived with an egg or sperm from another person, we poor mortals have done all that man and God might expect of us.

Matters become more complex when a surrogate mother is involved. There, a woman is inseminated by a man so that she may bear a child to be delivered to another couple. That process uses a woman's body from the start for purposes against which her own instincts, as well as our own moral judgment, rebel.

The case of Baby M in New Jersey began with a child born in 1986 to a woman, Mary Beth Whitehead. She had entered into a contractual agreement with William and Elizabeth Stern to deliver the child to them. Mrs. Whitehead had become pregnant through artificial fertilization by Mr. Stern's sperm. After the baby's birth, Mrs. Whitehead refused to surrender it; the Sterns sued. The trial court judge decided that the contract should be honored and the baby should go to the Sterns. On appeal, the New Jersey Supreme Court unanimously decided that the contract was invalid but gave the baby to Mr. Stern (it was his sperm) and allowed Mrs. Whitehead visiting rights.

The contract, according to the court, was invalid because it violated the law and public policy of the state. It illegally used money to procure a child. More important, because no woman before the birth of a child can truly give informed consent to relinquishing an infant she has borne and seen, Mrs. Whitehead had not entered into a valid contract. At that time, and so far as I know, even today, in every state but Wyoming, no woman can agree to allowing her child to be adopted unless that agreement is ratified after birth. That had not happened in the case of Baby M.

Why, then, did the court give the child to Mr. Stern? For no good reasons, I think. The court did not like Mrs. Whitehead. She was poor, ill-educated, frequently moved, received public assistance, and was married to an alcohol abuser.

To me, Mrs. Whitehead's condition was largely irrelevant. The central fact was that she was the baby's mother; she was attached to it, even if it meant losing her fee. In a brilliant retelling of the case, anthropologist Robin Fox makes clear that the overwhelming body of biological and anthropological evidence supports the view that women become deeply attached to their children. The mother-child bond is one of the most powerful in nature and is essential to the existence, to say nothing of the health, of human society. I recount some elements of that bond in *The Moral Sense* and need not repeat them here. Though there have been academic squabbles about how best to measure the bond, there is very little disagreement that it exists.

In my view and, I think, in Robin Fox's, both courts were wrong. The child belonged to its mother, period. That does not mean that all forms of surrogate mothering are wrong, but it at least means that the buyer of the surrogate's services is completely at risk. Unless the surrogate consents to the adoption of the baby after it is born, the contract is invalid. Given that risk, surrogate motherhood will be unlikely, but it will occur in some cases. Some critics of my view would say that surrogacy is appropriate if the birth mother receives both egg and sperm from the parents who are to own the child. That mistakes genetic similarity for the birth effect. Mothers bear children and usually want them whatever their genetic origin. Parental investment is at least as important as genetic investment in explaining the bond between offspring and parents.

My views on assisted reproduction do not coincide with Dr. Kass's because I do not attach the same overriding significance to ordinary coitus as the source of children. I know of very little evidence that assisted reproduction, other than reluctant surrogacy, harms either the children or their parents.

Those considerations, of course, do not settle the matter of cloning. A powerful part of Dr. Kass's essay dwells on the origins of the egg. I am as repelled as he by the prospect of a family seeking to produce a copy of Wilt Chamberlain or Marilyn Monroe. (The reader can tell how old Dr. Kass and I are by the examples we pick.) Nor do I much care for the idea of taking eggs from a Nobel Prize winner.

But I disagree that the source of the embryo will powerfully alter how the child is raised or with whom it will form attachments. A female child cloned from its mother will not form a sexual relationship with her father, nor will a brother cloned from its father seek a sexual relationship with its sister. When children grow up, they resist sexual attachments to those people whom they know best—that is, with whom they grew up. This is the reason that raising baby girls and baby boys from different parents together on an Israeli kibbutz does not make the grown-up girls and boys marry one another.

Limits on Cloning

I certainly favor limiting cloning to intact, heterosexual families and placing sharp restrictions on the source of the eggs. We do not want families planning to have a movie star, basketball player, or high-energy physicist as an offspring. But I confess that I am not clear as to how those limits might be drawn, and if no one can solve that puzzle, I would join Dr. Kass in banning cloning. Perhaps the best solution is a kind of screened lottery akin to what doctors performing in vitro fertilization now do with donated sperm. One can match his race or ethnicity and even select a sex, but beyond that he takes his chances.

Given those restrictions, why clone at all? The limited argument in favor of it arises from circumstances in which the husband and wife cannot conceive a child, in either the uterus or the petri dish. Cloning would thus be a substitute for either adoption, surrogate motherhood, or in vitro fertilization using cells from an unknown donor. The cloned cell would come from a friend or extended family member, thereby reducing the degree of genetic uncertainty that artificial insemination with sperm from an unknown donor produces.

I am persuaded that if only heterosexual families can clone, and if we sharply limit the sources of the embryo they can implant in the woman, cloning will be quite rare. Sex is more fun than cloning, and artificial insemination and in vitro fertilization preserve the element of genetic chance that most people, I think, favor. Dr. Kass is right to stress the mystery and uncertainty of sexual union. That is why hardly any woman with a fertile husband who could obtain a sperm from a donor bank will do so. Procreation is a delight.

About the Authors

Leon R. Kass is the Addie Clark Harding Professor in the Committee on Social Thought and the College of the University of Chicago. He is the author of *Toward a More Natural Science: Biology and Human Affairs* and *The Hungry Soul: Eating and the Perfecting of Our Nature.* Professor Kass is an adjunct scholar of the American Enterprise Institute.

James Q. Wilson is the James A. Collins Professor of Management and Public Policy Emeritus at the University of California, Los Angeles. He is the author of *Crime and Human Nature* (with Richard J. Herrnstein), *Thinking about Crime, On Character, The Moral Sense,* and *Moral Judgment.* Professor Wilson is chairman of the Council of Academic Advisers of the American Enterprise Institute.

A Note on the Book

*Leigh Tripoli of the publications staff of
the American Enterprise Institute
edited this book. Alice Anne English designed
this book and set it in the typefaces
Bembo and Zapf Chancery.
Edwards Brothers, Incorporated, of Lillington,
North Carolina, printed the book on
permanent acid-free paper.*

The AEI Press is the publisher for the American Enterprise Institute for Public Policy Research, 1150 Seventeenth Street, N.W., Washington, D.C. 20036; *Christopher DeMuth,* publisher; *Dana Lane,* director; *Ann Petty,* editor; *Leigh Tripoli,* editor; *Cheryl Weissman,* editor; *Alice Anne English,* production manager.